SO-AUX-026

STOMACH ULCERS AND ACIDITY

Explains the causes of these common complaints
and shows how to avoid and treat them.

THE NEW SELF HELP SERIES

STOMACH ULCERS AND ACIDITY

PRACTICAL MEASURES TO HELP YOU AVOID AND TREAT THESE PAINFUL STOMACH DISORDERS

LEONARD MERVYN
B.Sc., Ph.D., C.Chem., F.R.S.C.

THORSONS

THORSONS PUBLISHING GROUP

First published in *The Science of Life* series

This edition published 1990

© THORSONS PUBLISHING GROUP 1990

British Library Cataloguing in Publication Data

Mervyn, Leonard, *1930*-
The new self-help stomach ulcers and acidity.
1. Man. Gastrointestinal tract. Ulcers. Therapy. Self-help
I. Title
616.34306

ISBN 0 7225 2257 6

Published by Thorsons Publishers Limited,
Wellingborough, Northamptonshire, NN8 2RQ, England.

Printed in Great Britain by
William Collins, Sons & Co. Ltd, Glasgow

1 3 5 7 9 10 8 6 4 2

Contents

Note to Reader

Foreword

Stomach and duodenal ulcers occur as a culmination of rejecting Nature's warnings over a period of years. Ulcers in either the stomach or duodenum don't just happen, they are often the result of years of wrong eating habits, worry or stress, or failure to cope with our modern lifestyle and ignorance concerning how our body functions and how we can best look after it.

Man was never intended to live in our huge 'civilized' cities in an environment which is foreign to his 'natural' habitat. For centuries, in our Western civilization, man lived in a rural or semi-rural atmosphere. Even the big cities of 100 years ago were small in comparison to the sprawling metropolises we know today. During the past fifty or sixty years life has become much more complex, complicated and hazardous as we continue to make what we choose to call 'rapid progress'. No longer do we obtain fresh milk direct from the dairy, but in bottles or cartons which may be a few days old or, if it has been subjected to ultra high temperature processing, it may be several months old. We eat more processed, ready prepared and take-away foods. In Australia one leading dietitian has said that 'one third of all meals are prepared or eaten away from the home and the public don't know what they are getting'. On top of this government statistics show that 25 per cent of all kilojoules (calories) available to the Australian public come from alcohol or sugar. It is little wonder then that we see an ever increasing incidence of stomach and digestive disorders. Our food is not what it used to be and consequently we have paid the price of deteriorating health.

Not all progress is bad, however, and if we can adjust our way of living and our way of thinking to accommodate change we can do much to reap the benefits offered by our modern civilization without losing our health or the quality of life we have been accustomed to enjoy.

Stomach ulcers are usually carefully nurtured and grown with loving care by the sufferer who is usually totally ignorant of what he is doing. Before an ulcer develops there are usually warning signs, digestive upsets and minor discomfort for months and very often for years before the ulcer becomes apparent. It is by paying attention to Mother Nature's warning signs and by successfully overcoming minor digestive problems that more serious disorders including gastric and duodenal ulcers can be avoided.

The digestive tract can be broadly divided into four sections. There are the mouth and oesophagus (gullet), the stomach, the duodenum and small intestine and the colon or large bowel. The chemistry of these four sections varies alternately from alkaline to acid. The mouth and oesophagus are alkaline, the stomach is acid, the duodenum and small intestine are alkaline and the colon or large bowel is acid. It is imperative that each section maintains its normal alkalinity or acidity for normal digestion and that each stage of digestion be satisfactorily completed before the food passes to the next section for further processing.

Digestion begins in the mouth and if food is not chewed thoroughly and completely mixed with saliva before passing to the stomach, digestion in the stomach is impaired. Anyone who suffers with any digestive problem should chew their food for at least twice as long as they are accustomed to do. Remember that you cannot overchew your food. Eat at a leisurely pace and chew it well.

Food transit time through the digestive system is also important. The food only remains in the mouth for a few minutes. In the stomach it takes from 2½ to 5 hours before the food is ready to pass to the duodenum. It takes a further 3½ to 4½ hours for the food to pass through the duodenum and small intestine before it reaches the large bowel. It should then pass through the large bowel in another 12 to 15 hours making a total transit time of about 20 hours. In our Western diet with its predominance of refined carbohydrates, alcohol, sugar and fat transit time can be as long as 72 hours! This means that many toxins from waste products can be reabsorbed into the system giving rise to all manner of illnesses. It is also important to realize that over 90 per cent of nourishment from our food is absorbed from the first half of the small intestine, some 3 to 5 hours after we have eaten it. Little absorption occurs after the food has proceeded past this point.

Food transit time is influenced largely by the type of food we eat and also by exercise. Physical exercise is essential to normal digestion and it is usually sedentary workers who suffer with digestive problems although manual workers are not immune from them, particularly if they eat their food quickly, wash it down with tea or coffee and visit the local pub regularly after work. To maintain normal food transit time adequate fibre must be included in the diet, so too must a plentiful supply of fluids, preferably water. It is unwise to drink with meals. Most people who drink with meals do so because they fail to chew their food thoroughly and so have to wash it down instead of mixing it with saliva and enabling it to slip down the gullet easily. Drink twenty minutes after a meal, not while eating.

Our Western diet also contains an excess of fat, sugar and salt. These should be reduced but not excluded from the diet. Stimulants such as tea, coffee and alcohol should be avoided.

What happens once an ulcer has developed? How do we overcome it and prevent it from recurring? That is just what this book is all about. There are many simple, easy-to-follow measures which can be employed to assist ulcer sufferers. Correct diet, simple herbal remedies, overcoming stress and learning to live in our present day environment are all important to the ulcer sufferer. The value of foods such as yogurt, herbs like slippery elm bark and liquorice, vitamins and minerals are all explained simply and clearly. If you do not have an ulcer this book will show you how to avoid it; if you are unfortunate enough to suffer with one then this book contains much valuable information to help you overcome it.

1

The Digestive System

Before we consider and discuss the various aspects of gastric and duodenal ulcers it is important to understand the whole process of food digestion. Not only is food subjected to a superbly controlled sequence of processing from the time it enters the mouth to its eventual excretion; at each stage digestive juices of the right type and make-up play their part in reducing the food to a form in which it can be absorbed and utilized by the body. We need a digestive system because food constituents as presented in the diet are complex substances that have to be reduced to simpler ones before the body can assimilate them. Basically, during the process, starches and sugar are digested or hydrolysed to the simplest sugar glucose. Proteins are reduced to their individual amino acids, some twenty or so in all. Fats and oils are emulsified then broken down to their constituent fatty acids and glycerol, which are partially re-combined after absorption to produce the type of fats that the body needs. Some of the glucose remains to be used as fuel for the workings of the body but most of it is built up into animal starch called glycogen which forms part of the fuel reserves, ready to be split once more into glucose when required.

The amino acids derived from the food are absorbed as such then combined by body processes to produce the proteins specifically for the human body. Some amino acids are set aside for other uses, for example, as brain and nerve transmitters; others can be utilized as fuel and inter-converted to make other amino acids. Fats represent a very important energy reserve since they are readily broken down and fed into the energy-producing cycle, like glucose, but they do have other specific functions. These are usually well catered for so that the problem is usually too much rather than too little fat laid down as energy storage depots.

It is relatively easy to break down the basic food constituents in the laboratory or in a factory. Boiling starches and proteins with acid will produce glucose and amino acids respectively. Boiling fats and oils with alkali will yield the free fatty acids (as sodium salts) and glycerol as in making soap. The digestive process is much less drastic although the end results are the same.

The body utilizes enzymes that are specific protein (organic) accelerators or catalysts that under certain conditions will break down the food constituents just like acids and alkalis do but in a more gentle manner. These enzymes require other constituents and narrow limits of acidity and alkalinity to digest food efficiently and the digestive processes are geared to supply these. Of course, digestive enzymes despite being proteins in structure, are not affected by the conditions under which they act in the digestive tract but are usually de-activated as they move through with the food at the next stage.

We shall now look at the process of digestion as it occurs at the various levels of the gastro-intestinal tract. The first stage happens in the mouth but even before food is introduced into it, various stimuli have caused the digestive juices to be produced. Even whilst the meal is being prepared, the smell of the cooking food, the thought of the taste to come and the anticipation of satisfying the appetite causes the saliva to flow. At the same time gastric juices, very potent in acids and enzymes, are secreted. Lower down in the twenty-two feet of small intestine other juices are being produced in readiness for the anticipated food. Apart from salivation the most obvious sign of the approaching meal is the gurgling of the stomach juices although this can be a symptom of hunger even without food in the offing!

The Mouth
The saliva produced by specific salivary glands in the mouth is there to lubricate the food and assist in the actions of chewing, cleaning the mouth and swallowing. In addition it contains an enzyme, ptyalin, that converts starches into maltose, a sugar that is almost at the ultimate stage of digestion. There is some doubt regarding the signifi-cance of this early digestive process since starch is readily digested further down the system. The efficiency of ptyalin depends upon how long the food is chewed; in animals that bolt their food,

salivary ptyalin is absent.

The functions of the mouth and tongue are thus essentially to prepare the food for the main digestive processes further down the tract. They assist in the mastication of food and its formation into a bolus; they assist in swallowing. In addition the tongue is the sensory organ for the appreciation of taste, texture and temperature of food. Taste and texture are the stimuli to keep the digestive fluids flowing after their initial response to the smell of food.

These senses too are the first line of defence against eating food that is 'off'. The nose is the first to spot it and the usual reflex action is to spit out the obnoxious food. If some has already been swallowed both taste and smell will exert their protective actions by telling the stomach to refuse to pass the food on. The reverse process comes into play so the bad food is squirted back into the mouth from where it is readily vomited. The whole process is usually preceded by nausea so there is plenty of warning that the food is about to be rejected. Sometimes the food may have been passed on through the stomach to the intestine. This is usually the point of no return since there is a valve preventing intestinal contents from going back into the stomach. In such an instance the intestinal muscles will react by passing the poisonous contents quickly through the rest of the digestive tract. The end result is diarrhoea that disposes of the noxious material, eliminating it from the body. Hence although unpleasant, nausea, vomiting and diarrhoea are essentially protective and beneficial mechanisms.

The Oesophagus or Gullet

Although the oesophagus does not contribute to the digestive process, it links the mouth and the stomach. The walls of this connecting tube push the food into the stomach by a process of peristalsis which is simply alternating contraction and relaxation of the muscle. Gravity also contributes but peristalsis is the main process since thanks to this it is perfectly feasible to swallow when standing on one's head. There is some sort of valve, albeit not a very efficient one, between the oesophagus and the stomach so there is a little slowing down and control of the passage of food into the stomach. Usually however, the food passes fairly quickly into the stomach after swallowing. We shall see later how reverse movement of stomach contents into the oesophagus gives rise to a distressing condition called oesophagitis.

The Stomach

The stomach and the rest of the alimentary tract are shown in their relationships in Figure 1.

As the food is chewed the fluids produced by the salivary glands and the stomach continue to flow. The food is pulped with the teeth, tongue and the insides of the cheeks and mixed thoroughly with saliva. Eventually it is neatly packaged together at the back of the tongue where there are specific nerves that are stimulated to induce the act of swallowing. Once anything touches these nerves swallowing becomes an involuntary reflex action and nothing can stop the food or drink from entering the oesophagus.

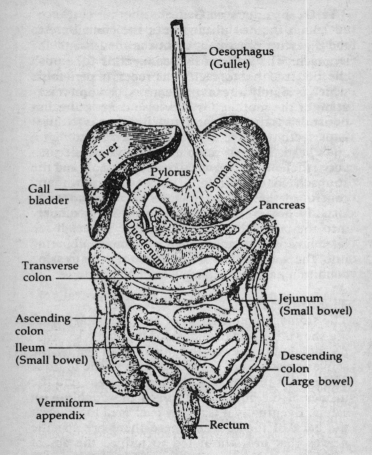

Figure 1. The digestive system

Note the length of the duodenum, the long, narrow neck which connects the stomach to the small intestine. About 75 per cent of ulcers occur in the duodenum.

Adjacent to the oesophagus is another entrance that leads down to the lungs or up into the nose. As food is swallowed a small soft body called the uvula rises to block off the nasal passages; at the same time the larynx (leading to the lung) is sheltered under the epiglottis so preventing food from entering the lungs. Food is thus directed down the oesophagus and as we have seen, it inevitably enters the stomach.

The stomach is of variable shape according to its contents and has the capacity to expand. It lies in the upper abdominal cavity, more to the right than the left. It is here that the digestive process really starts. Its action is like that of a washing machine where the pulped food gets turned over and over so that the various digestive juices can reach all parts of it. The walls of the stomach are rich in glands which secrete many substances. They include:

(a) Mucin, a protein that acts to protect the walls of the stomach from acid.

(b) Gastric juice which contains pepsinogen, which is inactive itself but is converted to the enzyme pepsin by another secretion, hydrochloric acid. Pepsin starts the breakdown of proteins. Another component, rennin, curdles liquid milk protein called caseinogen into the solid protein casein. This is then acted upon by pepsin.

(c) Hydrochloric acid which creates an acid environment essential for the digestive enzymes to work. At the same time this acid can disinfect the food destroying harmful bacteria. It also destroys ptyalin the salivary enzyme. Hydrochloric acid also controls the pylorus which is the valve that functions between the stomach and the next length of small intestine known as the duodenum.

(d) Hormones called gastrins are also secreted and they have the function of keeping up the flow of gastric juice until the meal is digested. Gastrins also stimulate the release of intrinsic factor from the stomach walls and as we shall see later, this factor is absolutely essential for the absorption of vitamin B_{12}.

(e) Lipases which help digest fats are also secreted in the stomach but their significance is doubtful since fat digestion is mainly the province of the intestine.

The stomach has a unique function not only as a processing chamber but also as a food store, for it has the capacity to expand to hold large quantities of food at a time. Drink that enters the stomach with food is passed on very quickly but some is mixed with the food, softening it further. Then it is squirted, a little at a time, into the next part of the gastro-intestinal tract, the duodenum. At this stage the stomach contents are known as chyme.

The Duodenum
The duodenum is about twelve inches long and is like a horseshoe in shape. It comprises the first part of the small intestine. It leaves the pylorus valve at the stomach and encircles the head of the pancreas to which it is firmly attached. It lies mainly to the right of the midriff and continuous to the next bit of the intestine called the jejunum.

The duodenum receives juices from two sources, the pancreas and the liver, via the pancreatic duct and bile duct respectively. Both juices are strongly alkaline so that in addition to their other functions they serve to neutralize the highly acidic chyme being squirted in from the stomach. The alkaline conditions that result in the duodenum act as the ideal medium in which the enzymes secreted in the duodenum can continue with the digestive process.

Pancreatic fluid is not only efficient in liquefying the partly digested proteins and the starches present in the food from the stomach but it has also the capacity to attack the fats in it. Bile assists in this because it contains bile salts, such as sodium glycocholate and sodium taurocholate, that emulsify fats and oils, rather like washing-up detergents that remove fatty residues from dirty plates.

The enzymes present in pancreatic secretion are:

(a) Trypsinogen, inactive until converted to the active enzyme trypsin. This digests proteins and partly-hydrolysed proteins almost to amino acids.

(b) Chymotrypsinogen, inactive until converted to the active enzyme chymotrypsin by the other enzyme trypsin.

(c) Amylase, a starch-splitting enzyme that converts both starch and glycogen (animal starch) almost to glucose.

(d) Lipase, a fat-splitting enzyme that causes hydrolysis of fat to fatty acids and glycerol. This enzyme is activated by bile salts which are produced in the liver and secreted in the bile.

(e) Carboxypeptidase, secreted as inactive pro-carboxypeptidase but produced by the action of the other enzyme pepsin. The end result of carboxypeptidase digestion is some amino acids and combined amino acids called peptides.

The Small Intestine

The duodenum takes up only the first twelve inches of the small intestine. The rest is made up of the jejunum which is eight feet long and the ileum which comprises the last twelve feet.

Digestion is completed by enzymes secreted in the intestinal juices which are produced by the glands of Brunner and of Lieberkuhn. These enzymes are:

(a) Aminopeptidase and dipeptidase which between them complete the digestion of proteins to simple amino acids.
(b) Disaccharidases which complete the digestion of the products of digestion by amylases (pancreatic enzymes) to glucose.
(c) Lipases that are specific for digesting complex fats like lecithin.

The small intestine, along its whole length, is also the main site for absorption of all the products of digestion which are now in a suitable state to be absorbed.

Hence the small intestine performs both digestive and absorption functions. It is often abused yet continues in its efficient manner. When we consider the hot spices; the unnatural cooked food; the over-cooked or even burnt food items; the pips, stones, bits of paper, coins, even fragments of broken glass that we present the gastro-intestinal tract with, it is a miracle that the small intestine continues to digest and absorb. It can be polluted with medicines, alcoholic drinks, drugs, and infective micro-organisms yet it still carries on.

In spite of these abuses the stomach and the small intestine and indeed the rest of the intestinal tract continue to work virtually twenty-four hours a day, churning up food, kneading it, mixing it with self-made juices, squirting it for hours on end until almost every constituent of the food has been reduced to its basics. These basics are glucose, amino acids, fatty acids, vitamins and minerals. The only constituent not reduced further is dietary fibre but even this has an important function, as we shall see later.

Absorption of these basic food constituents is an intricate process and the cells of the lining of the small intestine are particularly adapted for it. They comprise a highly specialized absorbing surface which is so finely and intricately folded that the total surface area is about that of two tennis courts! This is necessary because of the sheer volume of the food and digestive fluids passing down the small intestine. Every day we make almost three gallons of these fluids in order to digest our food and most of this volume has to be absorbed back into the body or we would die of dehydration. This is why we can continue to suffer from diarrhoea even after drinking nothing – in this case all the fluids are not absorbed. Persistent diarrhoea can be dangerous, particularly in babies and small children, because they are unable to replace the huge losses of water being excreted. This is why fluids are often introduced directly into the vein, to bypass the diseased gastro-intestinal system.

The stomach does not absorb anything apart from alcohol. This explains why the euphoric effect of alcoholic beverages is so rapid – absorption starts as soon as the stomach is reached. The ill-effects of alcohol appear much later because the body takes time to start disposing of the substance and it is the first metabolites like acetaldehyde that are toxic.

The Large Intestine

The large intestine, which is about six feet long, starts with the caecum which joins the end of the ileum at the ileocaecal valve. After this comes the ascending colon which bends at a right angle to continue as the transverse colon then turns through another right angle downwards to form the descending colon. The end of the colon (also called the large bowel) is the pelvic colon which joins to the rectum. This is the end of the line as far as food residues are concerned because the rectum ends in the anus, the excretory exit for the faeces.

The ileocaecal valve allows the food residues from the small intestine to go through into the caecum a little at a time. By this time the residues have less and less digestible material left with proportionately more of the indigestible plant fibre – cellulose and lignin – derived from fruit, vegetables and bran. In addition there is a very large quantity of bacteria present. These bacteria are the so-called 'friendly' ones that are beneficial to us, helping in the rotting-down process of the vegetable constituents in the food we eat. During this process they produce some B vitamins and the fat-soluble vitamin K. A proportion of these are absorbed so that we can make use of them and they contribute to our daily allowance of certain vitamins.

Strong antibiotics unfortunately kill these good bacteria, as well as the harmful ones, sometimes to such an extent that our intake of B vitamins and vitamin K is seriously reduced. For this reason these vitamins are sometimes prescribed with antibiotics. If they are not, it is still useful for an individual to take a vitamin B complex product whilst on antibiotics and for a short period afterwards. Destruction of 'friendly' bacteria can also cause diarrhoea so freeze-dried preparations of them in powder form or even living yogurt can help by supplying fresh colonies.

The food has been digested and its nutritious components absorbed by the time it reaches the beginning of the large intestine. It is still however semi-fluid and the function of the large intestine is to extract most of the remaining water. This conservation of water in our body is important since if it were allowed simply to go through the rest of the system, dehydration would soon result. The mass of food residue plus bacteria is steadily pushed along the large intestine, losing more and more water along the way, and finally ending up as a solid mass. In this form it is stored near the end of the large intestine where accumulation takes place before the final excretion.

This mixture is now faeces and at a certain time, usually after breakfast, it is transferred *en masse* into the rectum. The rectum responds by telling the brain that it wants to rid itself of this material and the end-result is the desire to defecate or 'open the bowels'. Under normal conditions this is complete. The semi-solid faeces are extruded in the characteristic sausage form which in fact reflects the shape of the lining of the rectum. The act of defecation to completion immediately produces a strange feeling of well-being and satisfaction. At the same time it must be remembered that this material is not normally poisonous or harmful. It consists mainly of undigested fibre and harmless bacteria that can continue this 'rotting-down' process even after leaving the body. The brown colour of normal faeces is derived from bile pigments – the smell comes from the decomposition process caused by the 'friendly' bacteria.

Although most of the food constituents of our diet are digested then absorbed, the undigested fibre plays an important role throughout the digestive tract. Because they cannot be digested, fibres such as these found in bran, fruit and vegetables survive throughout the whole system and add bulk to the food contents. This bulk enables the whole of the gastro-intestinal system to carry out its peristaltic action in moving the food, even when mainly digested, along the tract. At the same time, these fibres absorb water and in so doing they swell, giving the walls of the gut a solid mass to work on. At the excretory end fibre is really important since its bulk and water-retaining capacity enable the faeces to maintain a semi-solid state. Constipation is due to over-absorption of water resulting in hard, compacted faeces; diarrhoea is the retention of too much water by the faecal mass. Hence dietary fibre can help by normalizing the water content of the excreta in both cases.

It seems that even soluble, indigestible food fibres like guar gum and other vegetable gums have an important part to play in the absorption and excretory systems. When dissolved in water, these gums act like a gel which also supplies bulk to the food mass. As gels they perform two very important functions. They slow down the absorption of sugars, so preventing a massive rise in blood sugar occuring after a meal. In addition they retain water and hence present bulk to the faecal constituents, aiding the insoluble fibres in their functions.

2

Indigestion and Related Conditions

There are many conditions associated with the stomach and adjacent parts of the digestive tract that can be a prelude to or consequence of gastric ulceration and excess acidity. These can be prevented or treated by sensible eating and care in the diet. Knowledge and correct diagnosis of these conditions and their early detection and treatment can often prevent the occurrence of the more serious peptic ulceration and its consequences.

Simple Indigestion

Eating too much denatured and processed food, eating too quickly, and eating badly prepared or ill-assorted combinations of food, can all bring on an attack of acute indigestion. This is also known as dyspepsia but no matter what it is called, it causes much discomfort. Sometimes this is relieved by vomiting which is Nature's way of curing it. More often though there is a very unpleasant feeling of nausea. Relief can be gained by drinking heavily salted water or, more drastically, by sticking two fingers down the throat. These heroic measures are not often needed however. Relief is often obtained simply enough by getting some cool, fresh air on the face or having a drink of cold water. Many people will experience a bloated, distended feeling often amounting to pain. One common cause is the result of air swallowed during the meal but it may also be due to nervousness. A meal that has lasted too long is often the reason. The best relief, embarrassing as it may be, is often a good belch. An attack of hiccups, though perhaps just as embarrassing, is usually the end-result.

For these symptoms there are many traditional remedies that are helpful – amongst the most pleasantly effective are the liqueurs taken at the end of a banquet. Originally this was why they were produced and drunk traditionally at the end of a meal and all are based on natural aromatic oils. Orange, peppermint, aniseed and dill are amongst the most popular and effective plant oils. Such oils are known as carminatives and in the hands of the herbalist are used extensively in the relief of flatulence. No one is quite sure how these oils in liqueurs settle the stomach but the alcohol content plays no part. Relief from flatulence is just as easily obtained from peppermints, orange slices, root ginger or essential oils from these plants. Just as important as taking this treatment is the half-hour rest after a heavy meal. In babies, gripe-water has the same carminative effect and it is worth remembering that this remedy can be just as effective in adults.

These treatments are all natural ones; to attempt to deal with the condition by taking strong medicine or alkaline powder is not the way to clear up the trouble. The price of purchasing a little momentary relief by these means is to render yourself more and more open to future attacks. Such treatment merely treats the effect. It makes no attempt to remove the cause which lies largely in our traditional feeding habits.

Both rich meals and alcoholic drinks have a dehydrating effect, probably because, as we have seen, vast amounts of digestive juices are needed to cope with the food and the body will draw on its reserves of water to supply them. Alcohol, by virtue of its properties, will literally draw water out of the body tissues. The simplest remedy to ensure against suffering the day after over-indulging in food and drink is to drink not less than a pint of water before going to bed. This makes up the balance of the water previously lost and is the best natural treatment. As we shall see, however, it is simpler and better not to over-indulge but look more closely at what you eat and drink.

Occasional indigestion, particularly in the evening, can often be relieved by other natural means. Try getting extra sleep by going to bed early or getting up late. Take at least two hours exercise in the open by walking, golfing or gardening. Eat only light portions of food such as fish and fresh fruit. Carry on drinking large volumes of non-alcoholic drinks like natural, unsweetened fruit juices to keep down the calories but increase your vitamin C intake. In all circumstances avoid sleeping pills. Don't be misled by taking 'the hair of the dog' alcoholic drinks. This is a complete fallacy as it is now known that alcohol can only delay recovery. Give your digestive system a chance to recover — don't overload it with the very foods that caused the trouble in the first place.

There are always people who seem to develop indigestion easily and frequently, almost to the extent of daily discomfort. Often such attacks occur after consuming rich red wines, spices or citrus fruits. Although frequent attacks may give the individual the impression that there is something medically wrong, this is not often the case. It is a nuisance that can be prevented by sensible eating. It is often quite erroneously assumed by such individuals that they are allergic to these and other food items. Real food allergies are quite different and often result in copious vomiting, diarrhoea and skin reactions that give rise to blotchy, itchy rashes and patches. True allergy can make the unfortunate individual very ill indeed. Once allergies have been professionally identified, the only remedy is to avoid the food items causing them. Simple indigestion is only very rarely due to an allergy.

Nervous Indigestion
The simple indigestion discussed above can have a variety of causes including, as we have seen, allergies to food constituents. In addition to these physical causes however we must also add those due to psychological trauma. In this case nervous tension is often the culprit; a condition that can be brought on by stress, worry, external pressures or even an imminent examination, interview or some other event. Too often the immediate treatment is to take sedatives and tranquillizers to calm the nerves since these are the basis of the problem. This approach is most unwise since these drugs only create much

worse problems of drug dependence, depression and drowsiness which in turn dulls the mind. Look instead to the cause of the nerviness. Self-examination may often be sufficient to rectify it. If you feel the need of a calming-down agent, seek a herbal preparation or a high potency vitamin B complex formulation. These are mild, safe, non-habit forming and function through natural methods on the nervous mechanisms.

When we consider that we do not consciously tell our digestive system to work it is obvious that to a large extent the nervous control of the whole digestive process is not under our own control. Nevertheless since nervous indigestion is a fact of life conscious thought can stimulate the flow of juices, perhaps when we don't need them, and contractions of the stomach and the rest of the digestive system. The nerves that tell our system these things reside in a large, multi-functional nerve called the vagus. This supplies many other organs of the body as well as the digestive tract so it is not surprising that mental factors can affect the workings of the stomach. In fact, one treatment for over-production of stomach acid and chronic indigestion is by cutting the vagal nerves that supply the stomach but this drastic therapy is now often replaced by less invasive treatments.

Chronic Indigestion

Many attacks of indigestion are temporary and giving the stomach a rest is often all that is needed for relief. Some people, however, do appear to suffer a constant discomfort after eating. This may be related to habitual wrong feeding and is aggravated rather than helped by the taking of one or more of the patent medicines on the market. Treatment therefore resides in a change in diet and it is gratifying to see how often this does the trick. This approach is dealt with later in the book but if, despite sensible eating, chronic indigestion persists it is sensible then to seek professional medical advice.

Heartburn

This is due to the acid stomach secretions regurgitating into the gullet, giving a burning sensation. This reflux of the stomach contents often happens when one is lying down after a heavy meal or even by bending down. Such heartburn is not unusual since it is simply related to the position of the body but if it happens in the upright position it means that the contractions of the stomach are actually pushing the acidic contents up into the gullet. They have managed to force their way through the ring of muscle between the gullet and stomach which, although not quite a sphincter or valve, usually manages to contract to hold the juices back. Although the stomach has an internal surface able to cope with acid, the oesophagus does not and it reacts by causing pain and burning sensation. The pain is known as heartburn and it is quite descriptive since it is frighteningly similar to the pain of some heart attacks. Again, if it happens only occasionally it may pass or it can be treated with a natural oil like peppermint but if it occurs consistently it should be treated by other means. It can be the cause of a disease called oesophagitis (see page 35).

People who are overweight have a greater tendency to suffer from heartburn. It can also happen in those with a malformation at the lower end of the gullet so that some of the stomach lies in the chest. This is called a hiatus hernia (see page 38).

'Indigestion' due to Wind

Whenever food, liquid or simply saliva is swallowed air usually accompanies it. This is just ordinary air that happens to be in the mouth at the time of swallowing. There is vast individual variation in the amounts of air swallowed; some people swallow several gallons during the course of a day. Even new-born babies swallow air. At birth there is no air in their stomachs but it is introduced as soon as they are able to swallow. Suckling is notorious for introducing air into a baby's digestive system resulting often in pain and discomfort that can only be relieved by a burp.

Usually we do not notice swallowed air but you can guarantee that it is always there. Only when it reaches large volumes does it become uncomfortable producing a relieving belch. The problem is that we invariably swallow more air in preparing to belch, only to bring it up again.

Too often, it is possible to get into the habit of associating the occasional ordinary feeling of mild discomfort in the stomach with 'a little bit of wind'. Attempts to belch it up cause more air to be swallowed, more discomfort and the whole cycle to start again. The end result is a glorious belch that was totally unnecessary in the first place as air was introduced as a deliberate action. Ignore ordinary, occasional mild twinges in the abdomen and don't exacerbate the condition by introducing unnecessary air.

It is amazing how often it is believed that 'wind' forms in the stomach. It does not. All air within the gastro-intestinal system has been swallowed. One of the most common abdominal complaints in the world is that of 'wind' but it is not a disease and singly reflects the bad habit of swallowing air. Belching may be considered a compliment to the chef in some parts of the world but it never justifies a visit to a practitioner nor does it indicate a dietary or digestive disorder.

Oesophagitis

Oesophagitis (inflammation of the oesophagus or gullet), gastritis and peptic ulcers are responsible for the vast majority of indigestion pains and difficulty in swallowing. We shall therefore consider each in turn but diagnosis of each particular complaint must be left to the practitioner.

The oesophagus is ostensibly a very simple structure but its mobility is similar to that of the gastro-intestinal system. At the top end it has a sphincter (or valve) that acts as a barrier to accidental swallowing because it is usually constricted, except when swallowing. The lower sphincter, connecting with the stomach, is less well defined but it is a barrier sufficient to prevent continual reflux (bubbling up) of gastric contents into the bottom end of the oesophagus. It is more of a kink than a developed valve but combined with a slightly higher pressure in the oesophagus it usually prevents regurgitation of stomach contents.

The lining of the oesophagus simply provides mucus to lubricate swallowing, rather like saliva does in the mouth. Although the lining of the lower end may secrete a tougher mucus to stand up to acid gastric contents it is not able to withstand them for long and the burning pain of oesophagitis is due to a direct action of this acid on the lining of the oesophagus.

The oesophagus is a relatively simple structure and there are only a limited number of mechanisms operating in its disorders. The most usual are physical obstruction, an inefficient valve, direct damage and bleeding. Obstruction may be caused by a foreign body; a growth; muscular uncoordination of the valve; a spasm or by a stricture or narrowing of the tube due to scar tissue from a previous injury. Sometimes the valve fails to relax or open and when this happens the main symptom is difficulty in swallowing.

An inefficient valve will allow the gastric contents to squirt up into the oesophagus, causing inflammation and pain. Damage to the oesophagus can be caused by swallowing any corrosive substance or, in some cases, medicinal drugs. The antibiotics tetracyclines, the anti-spasmodic drug emepronium bromide, and the mineral supplement ferrous sulphate are the main offenders but there are other drugs that can cause a similar inflammation if incompletely swallowed. Bleeding in the oesophagus can be due to a variety of causes but the most likely is scarring of the lining with sharp foods like crisps, crushed boiled sweets and the like. Oesophagitis is made worse by smoking and drinking alcohol. Coffee and popular drugs like aspirin can also exacerbate the condition.

Signs and Symptoms of Oesophagitis: The two predominant symptoms of oesophageal disorders are difficulty in swallowing and pain. The cause of the pain is usually mucosal inflammation and is usually described by the sufferer as indigestion or heartburn. The pain is usually located behind the breastbone but it can radiate into the arms or neck. It is usually associated with meals or with certain foods; with posture, being intensified by bending forwards or lying back, and with the sensation of regurgitation, perhaps even into the mouth. These signs and symptoms are characterisitic of the condition 'reflux oesophagitis'.

If the pain is due to oesophageal spasm it is much less characteristic and more easily confused with the pain of a heart condition. It is, however, relatively rare. Loss of appetite and possibly nausea may also result from pain in the oesophagus, no matter what is the cause.

Bleeding from the oesophagus is very rare. However, any vomiting of blood is serious and requires medical attention. Unchanged blood, red in colour, suggests the origin of the bleeding is the oesophagus. On the other hand, partly digested blood that is colourfully described as 'coffee grounds' suggests it has arisen in the stomach or duodenum.

Difficulty in Swallowing (Dysphagia)

We have all experienced 'a lump in the throat' for emotional or other reasons and it makes swallowing difficult, uncomfortable or even painful. Anxiety and depression can cause the same sort of feeling and is often the reason for the 'relaxed throats' that are common in tense or nervous people. If the oesophagus is blocked or paralysed by disease however, it is possible to swallow quite easily but instead of carrying on down, the food stops moving and may be regurgitated into the mouth. Although sometimes secondary to pain, this type of difficulty in swallowing may be due to more sinister causes and professional help should be sought.

Hiatus Hernia

Hiatus hernia is a distinct anatomical defect where the sphincter between oesophagus and stomach is displaced from its normal site at the point level with the diaphragm where the oesophagus joins the stomach (see Figure 2). There are two types of hiatus hernia, the sliding type and the para-oesophageal type. These are also illustrated in the diagram.

In the sliding type of hernia, the top end of the stomach has slid up into the chest. The oesophagus empties into it perfectly well since the sphincter is well into the chest. Food goes down inside the gullet, past the diaphragm muscle and on into the intestine perfectly easily. The only discomfort in some people is that there is easy regurgitation of food back into the gullet from the stomach. The result is an acid heartburn pain just behind the breastbone after meals.

This sort of hernia is a minor problem and treatment of it is easy. If it is due to overweight, the painful regurgitation will stop once the individual loses weight. The reason is that once this happens the pressure inside the abdomen will no longer tend

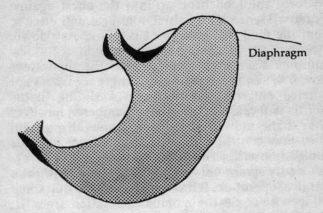

A para-oesophageal hernia

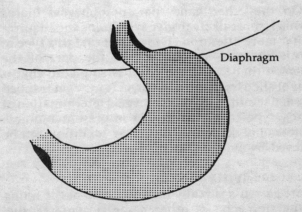

A sliding hiatus hernia

Figure 2. Types of hernia

to force the food back up into the chest against gravity. Hence all meals should be small ones so that the food will go down easily and stay down. Another tip is to stay sitting upright for a few minutes after each meal so that the food stays down. When these relatively simple measures are carried out, the discomfort of a sliding hiatus hernia will cease. It must be remembered however that if the individual is of a nervous disposition they may continue to suffer from simple nervous indigestion as described above. Sliding hiatus hernia is usually symptomless and hardly ever requires a surgical operation. It has been calculated that some 30 per cent of the population suffer from it. Sensible eating habits are still the best and easiest way to control the condition.

On the other hand, para-oesophageal hiatus hernia is more likely to give symptoms and requires rather more attention. The reason that this type of hernia is more serious is that the part of the stomach that lies in the chest is so placed that it cannot slide freely up and down. It may get trapped and hence suffer serious damage. Determination of which type of hiatus hernia is present requires professional diagnosis but either condition can be relieved by simple diet.

Acute Gastritis

Acute gastritis is really inflammation of the lining of the stomach. Its other name is acute erosive gastritis. It is usually caused by ingestion of alcohol, aspirin or other drugs, food and drug allergies or toxins from staphylococcal food poisoning. Sometimes the condition accompanies such apparently unconnected diseases like those of the kidney and infections like influenza. Other causes include, over-eating, the unwise combination of foods, or one or more of the dietetic indiscretions listed in this book. Usually gastritis is the stomach's definite indication that it can no longer tolerate the foolish and indiscriminate manner in which it has been fed and treated. It then proceeds to stage a strike against all further food until the whole digestive tract has been cleaned out – which is a somewhat painful and exhausting procedure.

Symptoms of acute gastritis are commonly lacking but loss of appetite, nausea, vomiting and gastric pain after eating may be present. Very occasionally the stomach lining may actually bleed. Treatment is usually aimed at withdrawing the offending agent, whether it is a medicinal drug or an allergic food. Changing the diet or ceasing to take alcoholic drinks will also relieve the condition. Fortunately the lining of the stomach regenerates itself very rapidly. Once the cause has been identified and removed, the self-healing process takes over and the stomach returns to normal after one or two days.

Corrosive Gastritis

This complaint is usually caused by swallowing strong acids, strong alkalis, concentrated iodine, potassium permanganate solutions or heavy metal salts like lead, mercury and cadmium. Gastric damage varies depending upon the nature and amount of the ingested poison. Often ulceration of the lips, tongue, mouth and throat will give a clue to the cause of the condition. Dysphagia or difficulty in swallowing suggests the oesophagus has also been damaged. The main symptom is severe abdominal pain sometimes accompanied by gastric bleeding.

The antidote and treatment depend upon the specific agent and amount taken and on the time interval before treatment. Acids are neutralized by alkalis and vice versa so here the antidote is fairly obvious. Other poisons may need expert advice, however, since induction of vomiting which may appear obvious may simply transfer the poison from the stomach to the gullet, throat and mouth where its corrosive action continues.

Chronic Gastritis

This is where the lining of the stomach is persistently inflamed but no one is quite sure what the cause is. Recent evidence suggests that the passing back or reflux of bile into the stomach is to blame. The bile acids have been particularly implicated in the condition since these are known to cause erosion of the stomach lining. Chronic gastritis is often a feature of gastric ulceration and in some cases may be the cause. Hence the dietary suggestions to prevent and treat gastric ulcers that are discussed later (page 118) should also help in overcoming chronic gastritis. Apart from dietary treatment there is no other effective therapy for this distressing condition.

Dyspepsia

Dyspepsia is a condition in which the nerves of the

stomach inhibit normal digestion and cause stomach acidity. Flatulence and gas pains are common. The typical dyspeptic is a neurasthenic. That is to say, his digestive troubles arise out of his restless, unrelaxed nature. He eats without discrimination at irregular intervals, leads a restless, ill-planned life, and subsists on a diet sadly deficient in all natural nerve foods and vitamins. He often smokes too much, drinks a lot of coffee, tea or spirits and fails to obtain sufficient sleep.

3

Peptic Ulcers, Their Symptoms and Causes

The number of people who suffer chronically from stomach or duodenal ulcers, acidity, dyspepsia or indigestion is appalling. No statistics are available, but unofficial estimates by medical men are to the effect that one person in every three over the age of thirty is either a chronic or partial sufferer from some kind of indigestion, gastric upset, or ulceration of the digestive tract. The pain and misery of these people as the result of their meals cannot be computed in terms of unhappiness.

It has been estimated that some twelve per cent of the adult population of Australia suffer from a stomach ulcer or its forerunner, chronic indigestion, after every meal. In Britain, medical authorities have estimated the number of sufferers from these two stomach ailments to be in the vicinity of four million. In the USA some authorities claim that as many as ten million people or more suffer from peptic or duodenal ulcers or acute, chronic indigestion. No club, no bar, no place where people meet is complete without its group of ulcer sufferers, and the doubtful humour which accompanies them. But ulcers are no joke. They are tenth among the list of chronic diseases as a cause of death and twelfth as a cause of absenteeism. American experts reckon that one out of every ten people is now bound to have a peptic ulcer sometime before they die.

Gastric ulcers occur mostly in early life. Duodenal ulcers usually pester middle age. Most ulcers are small – from a quarter of an inch to an inch in diameter. But they have an unpleasant habit of boring inwards through the walls of the stomach or duodenum rather than spreading along the surface. That's why ulcers kill. If they perforate those walls, you may die. Before we proceed, let us define the various types of ulcers to which human beings are vulnerable.

There are four times as many cases of stomach and duodenal ulcers among men than women, and for reasons which we will discuss later. The typical 'ulcer type' is generally lean, energetic, and anxious. Fat, placid men rarely get stomach ulcers. This is not to suggest that the lean, energetic type of person need get them – that to this type, stomach ulcers are inevitable. There is absolutely no need for any human being to become a victim of this painful – and highly dangerous – form of suffering that makes life a misery. Indeed, the suffering is incalculable, and the tragedy of it is that it is all so unnecessary. The consistent application of a few sensible principles can not only cure it, but can restore health to the highest level and keep it there.

What is a Peptic Ulcer?
Any ulcer is defined as an open, concave lesion of

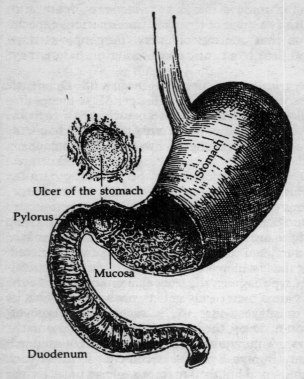

Figure 3. A stomach ulcer
An ulcer of the stomach, shown in the usual location,
just at the pylorus, or exit of the stomach. The duodenum
is shown below the stomach, and connects it with the
small intestine.

The stomach of the average human adult secretes
about three quarts of gastric juices daily. Gastric juices
contain hydrochloric acid, pepsin and rennin. These
digest food by chemical reaction.

varying depth in the skin or mucous membrane. In the case of peptic ulcers, they are erosions through the mucous membrane that lines the gastro-intestinal tract, penetrating the muscular layer and even the blood capillary bed. Although we associate peptic ulcers with the action of stomach acid eroding the membranes, the digestive or 'peptic' enzymes also contribute. Hence the term peptic ulcer applies to those found in the stomach itself (gastric ulcer); the first few inches of the duodenum (duodenal ulcer); the lower end of the oesophagus (oesophageal ulcer), and that formed at the sphincter between stomach and duodenum, called a pyloric ulcer.

All types of peptic ulcer are the result of acid and peptic enzymes. The acid is hydrochloric, a strong acid that is needed for digestion, for sterilizing food that may be infected or water that is contaminated. It is thus an essential secretion in our stomachs – later we shall see the serious consequences of the conditions where no acid is produced, known as achlorhydria. More likely, however, is the over-production of hydrochloric acid and hence the over-production of the peptic or digestive enzyme. What happens is that acid and enzymes leak back into the oesophagus causing ulceration. In the stomach, the most likely area for erosion by acid and enzymes is that of the lesser curvature of that organ. The most common form of ulcer however is found in the first inch or so of duodenum where the acid gastric contents first contact the duodenum lining. This lining is less resistant to acid than that of the stomach and erosion can take place before the alkaline secretions of the duodenum can effectively neutralize the acid gastric contents.

Peptic damage can vary widely in its effect. In its mildest form it may be present merely as inflammation, the best example of which is alcohol-induced gastritis. There may be small erosions most likely associated with certain drugs like aspirin and the anti-inflammatory medicines used in treating arthritis. The most severe form is a single large cavity that can reach half an inch in diameter, which is the classical peptic ulcer.

Since the gastro-intestinal tract has an inherent self-repair process, an ulcer is in a continuous state of flux with phases of damage and repair attending with each other. Examination by endoscopy (see page 52) hence reveals an inflamed active ulcer, full of exudate. In the quiescent repair stage that same ulcer appears as pale pink scar tissue.

The current view of peptic ulcer is that it is the result of an imbalance between normal erosive processes going on constantly and the ability of the tissue of the gastro-intestinal system to protect itself. Too much acid and digestive enzymes shifts the balance to the erosion side. In addition to these, however, must be included irritant drugs such as aspirin, anti-arthritic drugs, corticosteroids, iron salts, alcohol and bile. All of these can damage the lining of the stomach and duodenum.

What then are the protective factors? First and foremost is a thin layer of alkaline mucus secreted by the stomach lining. Production of this protective layer depends upon a healthy mucous membrane with the ability to have a fast turnover of cells to replace the inevitable losses. Replacement of these cells which produce the mucus, in turn depends upon various factors such as a good blood supply and protective hormones called prostaglandins. Both factors are the result of a good diet with an adequate supply of both vitamins and minerals so our food can play a big part in protecting us against peptic ulcers.

What are the Symptoms of an Ulcer?

The symptoms caused by ulcers are basically pain, the discomfort often making the sufferer belch as a result of trying to 'bring up the wind'. The pain is often quite characteristic in the way it comes and goes. Remember though that most instances of stomach pain have nothing to do with ulcers at all. These conditions were discussed in Chapter 2.

We have seen that the stomach can develop other disorders apart from ulcers even though the symptoms may be similar. The most common symptoms are loss of appetite, nausea, retching, vomiting and loss of weight. Even these can be due to emotional problems; disgust, for example, can easily cause nausea and vomiting; painful stomach cramps can arise from simple anxiety.

The usual symptoms of stomach ulcers are intense pain, vomiting, and occasional haemorrhage. The pain is the most consistent symptom, and may come on from half an hour to two hours after eating. Those with duodenal ulcers experience exactly the same symptoms, only in their case pain is felt a little to the right of, and above the navel, instead of in the stomach itself. There is usually a longer time lag between the meal and the pain.

Here are some of the many easily recognized
symptoms of ulcer:

- Chronic indigestion.
- Acid stomach.
- Acid belchings.
- Gas.
- Heartburn.
- Gassy distention.
- Burning sensation in the stomach.

In more severe cases these symptoms are present:

- Indigestion that appears about two hours after
  eating.
- Indigestion and stomach distress that suddenly
  stops when more food is eaten.
- Pain in the stomach.
- A sore spot in the stomach that is tender to
  pressure.
- Vomiting.
- Haemorrhage.
- Black-coloured stools. (They are black because
  of stomach haemorrhage.)
- Yellowing of the skin. (Caused by absorption of
  blood substance mixed in the food from bleeding
  ulcers.)
- Anaemia from loss of blood.

Of course, all of the symptoms may not be seen in
every case of stomach ulcer but any one is a very
suspicious indication that an ulcer is at work. Pain
after meals is the most common and most certain
symptom.

New York Specialist on Ulcer Symptoms

Dr Joseph F. Montague, a noted New York specialist, wrote the following useful outline of the symptoms of stomach ulcer and duodenal ulcer:

Stomach or duodenal ulcer starts a warning signal swinging in nine cases out of ten. That warning is pain, and the ulcer patient gets it invariably at some time of the day or night, if not at both of these periods, in the form of a sharp feeling of distress or a gnawing sense of discomfort. Whatever form the pain manifests itself in, it is well to heed it, for with ulcers generally an ounce of the good old prevention is worth the traditional pound of cure.

Very often when symptoms of so-called indigestion appear, the patient doses himself with this or that nostrum, or contents himself with taking a nightly purge. In the minds of many men there persists the belief that a physic will cure practically every ailment of the human body. So, the stomach ulcer patient, conscious of a burning sense of distress in his stomach, beneath his breast bone or between his shoulder blades, takes this or that laxative in the naive belief that he can wash his trouble out of him. Such purgatives are a positive menace where an ulcer is present, for they irritate tissue and stimulate peristalsis to a point that causes bleeding.

Duodenal ulcer, on the other hand, often has little effect upon the patient's weight. His appetite remains fairly normal and his only awareness of trouble in his digestive tract is the distress that comes along after he has eaten, or when he is about to eat again.

How Ulcers are Located

To find out if you have an ulcer, a doctor will

probably test the contents of your stomach before and after eating, and X-ray your stomach before and after you have eaten barium, which has a metallic content and therefore shows up on an X-ray photograph. If you have a chronic, deep ulcer the barium, an opaque substance, will fill up the hole the ulcer has left and reveal it. But it won't show up all ulcers, so your doctor may be left guessing whether that queer mark on your X-ray plate means that you have an ulcer or that you just have some kind of irritation.

With the increase of ulcer cases, medical science has devised a clever way of looking into the stomach. This is called cystoscopy. Scientists have produced a flexible tube with a system of lenses and electric lights and tiny mirrors which can be swallowed quite easily. It allows the operator to see inside the stomach, and even to take coloured photographs. A normal stomach has thick, smooth, orange-red folds. An ulcer looks like a small volcanic crater set in a red plush curtain!

Incidentally, most ulcers – three out of four – occur in the duodenum. The duodenum is the narrow neck of the stomach which connects it with the small intestine. Also, ulcers are more frequent among men than women, due chiefly to the fact that during their middle years, their stomach acid reaches a higher level. They eat more rapidly than women, and are likely to wash their meal down with tea, coffee, or beer, which are all acid-forming.

The Differences Between Duodenal and Gastric Ulcers

The causes of both types of ulcer are fundamentally different. Lack of the mucosal protection is the prime cause of gastric ulcers. When combined with irritation and inflammation of the stomach lining induced by various factors, a resulting ulcer is almost inevitable. The lack of a good blood supply to an area of the gastric mucous membrane also probably plays a part.

Duodenal ulcers are more likely to be a result of overexcretion of acid and peptic enzymes. The contact time between the duodenal lining and the erosive contents of the stomach as they pass into the duodenum also determines the susceptibility to duodenal ulcers. This can be prolonged for a variety of reasons and the chances of ulceration are increased. The effect of chronic stress is associated more with the developement of duodenal than with gastric ulcers. Acute stress is more likely to cause gastric ulcers.

The pain of duodenal ulcers is often relieved by food; that of the gastric type is aggravated. Night pain is more a feature of duodenal ulcers. The development of cancer can be a feature of gastric ulcers but there is no association between it and duodenal ulcers.

Risk Factors for Peptic Ulcers

Stress remains one of the most important factors for the development of so-called 'acute stress ulcers'. The term embraces not merely psychological stress but also the metabolic stresses associated with severe illness, burns, surgery, and accidental injury, all of which can produce peptic ulceration as a secondary feature. Other factors include smoking, group O blood, drugs, and a family history of gastric or duodenal ulcers. Although stress and medicinal drugs, because of their irritant action, may seem to be understandable factors, we are still uncertain as to why men are three times more prone than women to develop peptic ulcers. Nor do we understand why duodenal ulcers are three times as common as the gastric type. The fact that some five per cent of gastric ulcers become cancerous whilst duodenal ulcers rarely do is another mystery.

What are the Causes of Peptic Ulcers?

There are many causes, and most victims have for many years been guilty of not one, but several of the following:

- Over-eating
- Worry.
- The use of aluminium cooking utensils.
- Too much starchy food.
- Incompatible food combinations.
- Vitamin and mineral deficiencies.
- Mixed, messy and indiscriminate feeding.
- Hasty eating and improper mastication.
- Condiments
- Sugar consumption.
- The laxative habit.
- Alkaline powders.
- Weakened resistance of the blood to noxious bacteria.

These causes are not necessarily listed in order of importance, and generally a combination of several of them is responsible for the ulcer. Let us examine them in some detail:

1. *Over-eating:* Most people eat more food than they need for energy and the repair and maintenance of bone and tissue. All excess food puts an added strain on the digestive mechanism. Often it breaks down under the strain, and digestive troubles result.

2. *Worry:* The brain and the stomach are connected by the vagus nerve. Tests have shown that when a person is worried the flow of the powerful gastric juices in the stomach is increased. Indeed, under such conditions it continues to flow, whether food is present in the stomach or not. If there is the slightest ulceration in the stomach, the constant flow of the gastric juices – which contain hydrochloric acid – irritates the ulceration and enlarges it. On this point, Dr Richard Harrison has written:

> The stomachs of people with severe nerve weakness are in a constant state of irritation and unrest.
> This is because the nerves that stimulate normal stomach activity do not stop working when the stomach is empty.
> Instead, a continuous flow of irritating stomach juices is produced. On the walls of an empty stomach this continual, unnatural flow of stomach juices has a damaging effect.
> The stomach, after all, is a piece of meat. And stomach juices are designed to digest meat (and other protein foods).

Under ordinary conditions, Nature furnished good protection for the stomach tissues against its own juices. But when stomach tissues are continually saturated with a wholly abnormal amount of digestive fluid, some area loses the ability to further protect itself from damage ... An ulcer or ulcers is the result.

The destructive emotions of anger, rage, hate, jealousy and fear all have disastrous effects upon digestive processes. Meals eaten under mental or emotional tension lead to inadequate mastication, giving rise to faulty digestion. Worry and anxiety interfere with normal digestive activity.

3. *The Use of Aluminium Cooking Utensils:* Aluminium is a soft metal, readily affected when used for cooking foods because it is soluble in both acids and alkalis. Most foods have either an alkaline or acid reaction.

Traces of oxide of aluminium, when combined with sodium chloride (common salt) from the cooking of vegetables in salt water, and ingested with food, adversely affect the health-giving potassium in the human body. There is also evidence that these tiny particles of aluminium enter the stomach and weaken the stomach lining with their astringent properties, thus encouraging the formation of ulcers.

4. *Too much starchy (and protein) food:* Processed and refined starchy foods – bread, flaked, puffed and toasted cereals, porridge meals, cakes, pies, biscuits, rice, macaroni, etc. – constitute the bulk of the diet of the vast majority of the population. Both

processed, starchy foods and proteins are acid-forming and an excess of these foods in the diet upsets the proper acid-alkaline balance and leads to acidity – the forerunner of all digestive troubles (and, incidentally, of rheumatism and arthritis).

Alkali-forming foods, which are more desirable, include vegetables, fruits and most nuts, apart from Brazils and peanuts. Remember, however, that foods are acid- or alkali-forming only after absorption and assimilation by the body. Whilst in the digestive system, fruits, for example, contribute citric, malic and other acids. Although these are weak compared with the strong hydrochloric acid that the body produces itself, they do contribute some acidity.

The important point about food and the diet in general is to ensure that each meal is balanced. Food constituents themselves, particularly the proteins, have a neutralizing or buffering action on stomach acids that can help prevent the effects of over-production. There is no such action by starches and sugars.

5. *Incompatible food combinations:* Although a balanced meal, in respect of its various food constituents, is considered to be highly desirable by some authorities for the prevention of digestive problems this is not agreed by everyone. There is a modern school of medical thought which attributes much of the digestive troubles of men and women to the common practice of eating protein and starch foods, or acid and starch foods, at the same meal.

The starches referred to are – bread, packeted cereals, porridge meal, pastries, biscuits, jams, ice-cream, etc. These starch foods do not combine well in the stomach with protein foods (meat, fish, eggs and cheese) or with acid fruits (oranges, grapefruit, tomatoes, pineapples, peaches, plums, apples, apricots, etc.). This kind of 'incompatible feeding' often leads to gas, fermentation, flatulence, pain, and finally to chronic indigestion, dyspepsia, and/or ulceration.

The most sensible advice, however, is to be 'middle of the road' when it comes to eating meals, i.e. moderation in all things without excessive intake of any one particular food item, no matter how good you may think it is.

6. *Vitamin and Mineral Deficiencies:* It is no exaggeration to say that 90 per cent of the entire population suffers from vitamin and mineral deficiency of some sort. If this were not so, there would not be over 3,000,000 admissions to public and private hospitals every year in Australia, for example, and people would be far healthier.

In the case of digestive and ulcer sufferers, there is abundant evidence that these unfortunate people have long been deficient in vitamins A, B complex, C and E, and in calcium.

Vitamin A is required for the health of the epithelial tissue (i.e. the inside of the mouth, the tonsils, trachea, lungs, intestines, lymphatic glands, and the walls of the stomach, pylorus and duodenum). This vitamin has been shown in medical trials to be effective in accelerating the healing of peptic ulcers (see page 86).

The B complex vitamins are essential to the health of the nervous organization and the secretion of enzymes necessary for good digestion.

Vitamin C is required for healing any ulcer. Vitamin C builds healthy connective tissue and strengthens the walls of blood vessels. It also helps to stimulate 'antibodies' and phagocytes which destroy bacteria in the blood-stream.

Vitamin E acts most beneficially upon the heart and muscles. It dilates the capillaries and permits an improved flow of blood to congested areas. It also dissolves blood clots. Lack of this vitamin in the ordinary diet appears to have some bearing upon the increase in the number of stomach ulcers.

Calcium is important to the health of the body. Without it, the nerves and muscles cannot relax, giving rise to tension. Without Vitamin D (which we mostly obtain from sunshine) and phosphorus, the body cannot utilize the calcium in our food supply.

7. *Mixed, and indiscriminate feeding:* Most of us have grown up in the evil dietetic tradition that all so-called food is good for us – that it's all 'grist for the mill'. We therefore proceed to eat anything and everything that comes our way, regardless of the appalling task we have set our digestive organs, our eliminatory organs, and the chemistry of the body itself. Soup, meat, vegetables, puddings, washed down by tea or coffee – down it all goes! We may feel satisfied after such a meal but we have set in motion the ingredients which finally create fermentation, flatulence, acidity, hyperacidity, and stomach

trouble. If that were not bad enough, our next meal may add to the offence by consisting of one or other of the doubtful concoctions found in the delicatessen shop. Here we see a picturesque assortment of embalmed, preserved and demineralized products, masquerading as 'food' in the form of pies, pastries, pickled pork, pickled onions, corned beef, pigs' trotters, and an assortment of sausagemeats, consisting of meat scraps, flour, fat, colouring, and artificial flavouring and seasoning. All these products are alleged to feed you, but in reality they will hasten the onset of the pains of stomach ulcers and ill health.

A generation less notorious for its educated ignorance would condemn all such foods as unfit for human consumption. Very hot drinks, highly spiced foods and ice-cold drinks and foods all irritate the stomach lining. Sufferers from stomach troubles should also abstain from alcohol which increases the acidity of the stomach.

8. *Hasty Eating and Improper Mastication:* Every one must surely realize the digestive troubles they are inviting by eating meals under mental tension, leading to improper mastication and digestion. It is recognized by medical science that worry, anxiety and stress interfere with the normal activity of the stomach and that anger, rage and fear tend to over-excite and over-activate the flow of gastric juices.

9. *Condiments:* A further potent cause of ulceration is the habit of taking condiments. We have come to depend upon the artificial stimuli of mustard, pickles,

pepper, chutney, tomato sauce, salt, etc., to give us an appetite. But all these products are harmful irritants. They certainly stimulate appetite by exciting the flow of gastric juices but it is unnatural stimulation. The result is to leave the appetite more jaded than ever, so more stimulants are used, and so on. The result is that the lining of the stomach is subjected to such irritation that it becomes inflamed and finally ulcerated.

10. *Sugar Consumption:* Sugar, whether white or brown is a refined, concentrated carbohydrate completely divorced from all the beneficial elements of the original sugar cane. It is sweetness without sustenance, devoid of the essential vitamins and minerals. Molasses, the residue of sugar cane, has nutritional virtues. But sugar is left with only the dangerous delusion – the highly refined crystals that please the eye, seduce the palate and increase acidity. But in spite of its pleasant appearance and taste, sugar is a slow, insidious poison, robbing the body of its calcium by neutralizing it, setting up fermentation and acidity, and slowly but remorselessly undermining the health of its host. If you value your health, don't use sugar. If you want a substitute, use honey, which contains both vitamins and minerals.

At one time, it was usual to over-emphasize the factors of stress and strain as the dominant cause of stomach ulcers. However, research done in the 1960s showed that there are fewer ulcers among top-ranking businessmen than among lower paid people doing routine jobs. The survey found that shift workers in particular are very prone to ulcers.

It also revealed that there are more stomach ulcers among townspeople than country dwellers, not because there is more stress in town living, but because townspeople eat more sugar. Moreover, stomach ulcers are now not uncommon among children, doubtless due to an unbalanced diet containing a high proportion of sugary foods, refined cereals, soft drinks, sweets, ice-cream, chewing gum, etc. More attention than ever before is now being directed to faulty nutrition as the real cause of stomach ulcers.

11. *The Laxative Habit:* The taking of laxative pills and medicines is a notorious contribution to ulceration and inflammation of the digestive tract, especially the stomach. These laxatives are irritants; foreign bodies, which cause fermentation and unnatural stimulation of the nerves, muscles and mucous membrane of the stomach and alimentary tract. One authority explains their internal reaction as follows:

> When a purgative of any kind is introduced into the system, its presence is a constant irritation to the sensitive mucous lining of the bowel. The intestines react against the purgative, and in forcing it out of the system a bowel action necessarily takes place. But mark the fact that the action is brought about by the expulsion of the salts, or whatever it is, which the body regards as something foreign and repugnant to it.

It is now known that the regular use of laxatives can give rise to serious, even incurable, intestinal ailments in later years. Proper feeding will bring about regular bowel movements without pills or purgatives and the evils they lead to in the digestive system.

12. *Alkaline Powders:* Sufferers from digestive troubles or stomach ulcers usually seek refuge in one of the antacid powders or bicarbonate of soda preparations on the market. They feel that because these alkali powders give some relief from the pain and flatulence which follow every meal, they must be counteracting the acidity and so assisting in the healing of the ulceration. This is not the case, however. The antacid powder or bicarbonate of soda habit will in time make the condition worse. It does nothing to remove the cause of the trouble.

Dr William Howard Hay was once asked if antacid powder or bicarbonate of soda should ever be used to relieve indigestion or 'sour stomach' and he replied:

Not if used to correct stomach acidity, for it would aggravate the very thing for which relief was intended. Sour stomach comes from either an over-supply of hydrochloric acid or from the various fermentations of the carbohydrate foods (starches and sugars).

If from too much of the stomach acid mentioned, then correction by the soda merely means that enough or more of this acid will be secreted to continue the interrupted protein digestion, thus increasing the habit of formation of this, while if due to fermentation, this merely neutralizes the acids without in any way stopping the fermentation, which proceeds at the old rate.

The B complex vitamins, vitamin C, calcium, and iron, all need an acid medium in the stomach in which to carry out their various functions in promoting bodily health. Bicarbonate of soda, antacid powders and other alkalizers produce an artificially alkaline condition in the stomach, thereby neutralizing the action of the vitamins and minerals which are lost to the body.

13. *Weakened Resistance of the Blood to Noxious Bacteria:* This is the logical outcome of nutritional deficiencies and defects in the mode of life, so usual with the digestive and ulcer sufferer.

4

THE ROLE OF HYDROCHLORIC ACID

If you look up a chemistry text-book you will see hydrochloric acid described as a colourless fuming aqueous solution of hydrogen chloride gas with a very pungent odour. Yet this same acid in a dilute form is an important part of the human digestive system and its excess or lack can have profound effects upon the health of the individual. When too much is produced the condition is known as hyperacidity and this is one of the factors contributing to the formation of peptic ulcers. When too little is formed, the condition is called hypoacidity and the net result can be less effective digestion in the stomach. In some cases no acid at all is produced and the condition is referred to as achlorhydria. The absence of hydrochloric acid will increase the chances of developing gastric cancers.

Before we consider these various aspects of hydrochloric acid production, let us see how it is made within the stomach.

The Production of Hydrochloric Acid

In the lining of the stomach there are two types of secretory glands. One consists of a single layer of secreting cells known as chief cells which produce digestive enzymes. The other type of secretory gland consists of cells arranged in layers. They are known as parietal cells which secrete hydrochloric acid directly into the gastric glands and hence into the stomach. The mixed secretion is known as gastric juice. It is normally a clear, pale yellow fluid of high acidity, (between 0.2 and 0.5 per cent hydrochloric acid) but with 97 to 99 per cent water. Also present are the protective protein mucin, inorganic salts and digestive enzymes.

Hydrochloric acid is a combination of hydrogen ions (which determine acidity) and chloride ions. Hydrogen ions arise in the following manner. Carbon dioxide which is present in blood plasma as a normal respiratory component passes into the parietal cell. This cell has blood plasma on one side with the opening of the stomach on the other. Within the cell there is an enzyme, called carbonic anhydrase, which catalyses the reaction between carbon dioxide and water to form a weak acid known as carbonic acid. This is the same acid that is formed in carbonated drinks like lemonade. Because it is weak, carbonic acid readily dissociates into bicarbonate plus hydrogen ions. Bicarbonate cannot leave the parietal cell to enter the stomach but readily passes back the other way into the blood. The second component of hydrochloric acid, chloride, is always present in the blood (this is why blood tastes salty) and readily passes through the parietal cell and into the stomach itself. Here it combines with the hydrogen ions already produced by this specific cell and the net result is free hydrochloric acid.

Bicarbonate is alkaline and, as we have seen, this passes back into the blood. Hence after a heavy meal when hydrochloric acid is produced in great quantities, a lot of bicarbonate is also formed at the same time. This upsets the balance of acids and alkalis in the blood and it is then up to the kidney to restore the balance by getting rid of the extra bicarbonate into the urine. The end-result is the so-called alkaline tide which simply means that the urine is alkaline instead of slightly acid as normal. Alkaline urine promotes bacterial growth so too many 'alkaline tides' can eventually give rise to urinary infections.

Why do we Need Hydrochloric Acid?

This acid, along with some weaker organic acids that are also secreted into the stomach, provides the right sort of acidity that is essential for the first digestive enzymes to work. The digestion of proteins starts under the influence of the enzyme pepsin which cannot function unless the pH (measure of acidity) is between 1 and 2. Hydrochloric acid is essential for the gastric juices to reach this low pH (anything below pH7 is acid and the stronger the acid the lower the pH).

There is another enzyme, also secreted by the stomach, that requires a very acid medium in which to work. This is rennin and its main function is to coagulate milk into a solid form that can be acted on first by pepsin then by other enzymes further along the gastro-intestinal tract. Lack of hydrochloric acid will therefore make milk more difficult to digest.

It must be pointed out however that those people who have had the whole stomach, or just that part that produces acid, removed are still able to digest proteins and milk. Their digestive processes may not be quite as effective as they would be with a normally functioning stomach but it does suggest that the roles of pepsin and rennin are not quite as critical as was once thought.

The presence of hydrochloric acid, however, becomes of prime importance in the liberation of vitamin B_{12} from food and its eventual absorption. In meat, which is the most important provider of B_{12}, the vitamin is attached to proteins and the prior digestion of these proteins is essential for the vitamin to be released. Once it is free, vitamin B_{12} is able to combine with a specific protein called intrinsic factor that is also produced in the parietal cells of the stomach.

This complex of vitamin and intrinsic factor can only be formed in the presence of hydrochloric acid and calcium. Once formed, the complex is then transported intact to the ileum where it is absorbed. If intrinsic factor is not present, vitamin B_{12} cannot be absorbed and the result is the once-fatal disease called pernicious anaemia. Lack of hydrochloric acid will therefore reduce the absorption of vitamin B_{12}. It is not without significance that a major symptom of pernicious anaemia is a complete absence of hydrochloric acid in the stomach.

Increased Secretion of Hydrochloric Acid

We can now look at the factors that can cause an increased secretion of hydrochloric acid and its consequences. Of all the digestive tract, the stomach is one organ which is relatively easy to get at and its response can be studied by observing it in people who by reason of accident or design have a hole in the stomach, known in medical circles as a gastric fistula. The strength and quantity of hydrochloric acid produced by the gastric cells can thus be measured under a variety of conditions.

Psychological moods were found to be amongst the most influential factors in producing excess hydrochloric acid. Anger, worry and anxiety all caused the stomach walls to become red, swollen and inflamed with a marked increase in movement and gross over-secretion of acid. Other studies indicated that similar symptoms became apparent when the person was disgusted, resentful, depressed, fearful or when there was a reason to feel insecure, hopeless or defeated. Significantly, the recall of past frustrations or disappointments alone was sufficient to stimulate excess acid production.

As we have seen, hydrochloric acid secretion is usually the response of the stomach to an anticipated meal. The rumblings and gurgles associated with hunger are the stomach's reactions to the expected influx of food. Once it is eaten, though, the first-secreted hydrochloric acid is neutralized but secretion continues in order to maintain an acid medium.

Certain constituents of food have been found to be more stimulating to acid production than others. High protein foods like meat and fish, and beverages like coffee and tea all have a profound stimulant effect on acid secretion. Bitter materials have been known for years to have a stimulant effect on the appetite; now we know that aperitifs like sherry and campari simply act by causing hydrochloric acid to be produced.

Despite popular belief, highly spiced foods like chilli, curry, pickles, vinegar, soused herrings, mustard and frankfurters have little or no effect upon hydrochloric acid secretion. The burning sensation suffered by some people on taking these foods is more likely due to a localized effect of the 'hot constituents' on the lining of the stomach.

In view of the corrosive action of the highly acidic gastric juice, and the exposure of the stomach mucosa to it, perhaps it is surprising that this lining does not break down more often. If it does, of course, the result is a gastric ulcer. Usually, however, the stomach is able to protect its lining by secreting large quantities of mucus. This mucus forms a tough barrier and confers a high level of protection. It is quite possible that people who suffer from gastric ulcers produce only a thin, weakened type of mucus or possibly none at all.

Even when the ulcer has formed, if a thick layer of mucus covers it, it cannot be attacked by stomach acid and often the gastric lining is then able to heal itself effectively. A traditional remedy for treating gastric ulcers is liquorice and this has been found to act by stimulating the production of a thick layer of mucus over the area of the ulcer. A widely-used drug called carbenoxolone that is succesful in healing ulcers is derived from liquorice.

Other treatments for excessive hydrochloric acid production are simple neutralization with alkalis. Specific drugs and surgery are also used to control the acid production. Surgery involves cutting the nerve, called the vagus, which carries the impulses telling the parietal cells to make acid. Another approach is to use drugs that are known as histamine H_2 receptor antagonists. Since the naturally-produced histamine is a potent stimulator of hydrochloric acid production in the parietal cells, it is logical to use drugs that specifically block the action of histamine upon these cells. Hence acid production is curtailed and in its absence the irritant action is lost and the normal healing processes of the body are allowed to take over and get rid of the ulcer.

We shall see later how too little gastric hydrochloric acid can have serious consequences so it is possible that prolonged reduction in the secretion of acid by surgery or by drugs will increase the chances of these consequences. In a similar manner, constant neutralization of the stomach acid with oral alkalis can have serious effects: first by removing all of the acid so that the desired acidic medium in the stomach is lost; second because neutralization simply stimulates further production of acid so that more alkali must be taken and so on. A vicious circle is set up so that eventually the parietal cells simply give up.

Deficiency of Hydrochloric Acid
A deficiency or complete lack of stomach hydrochloric acid has more far-reaching consequences than an excess. Dietary minerals are solubilized by the acid and this makes them more amenable to absorption. Adelle Davis reported how an ortho-

paedic specialist found that his patients consistently
had low levels of hydrochloric acid. Once the
deficiency was overcome by supplementing with
the acid, the rate of bone healing and ossification
increased as more calcium became absorbed.

She also quoted references supporting the fact
that an insufficiency of hydrochloric acid can
result from a low intake of protein and deficiency of
vitamins A, B_1, B_2, B_6, niacinamide, choline and
pantothenic acid. Volunteers deficient in pantothenic
acid were found to have reduced hydrochloric acid
secretion as well as a decrease in digestive enzymes,
other digestive secretions and gastric motility. It
required three weeks of high potency treatment
with this vitamin before normal secretions and
motility were restored. Vitamin C absorption is
more efficient in the presence of hydrochloric acid
presumably because it keeps ascorbic acid in the
free form.

Achlorhydria

A complete lack of stomach hydrochloric acid
known as achlorhydria is a feature of several
diseases. The most common is chronic gastritis
where the parietal cells have been destroyed by
atrophy of the gastric mucosa. Cancer of the
stomach is usually characterized by achlorhydria,
mainly because the tumour envelops the parietal
cells so they no longer function. One of the diagnostic
features of pernicious anaemia is finding that there
is no hydrochloric acid produced. Even when the
anaemia responds to vitamin B_{12} injections, there
is no effect upon the gastric mucosa and hydrochloric

acid secretion is still curtailed. When the stomach is partially or fully removed by surgery, the source of hydrochloric acid disappears so that digestion can only start in the mildly alkaline conditions of the small intestine. In these circumstances and indeed in any other condition where achlorhydria is a feature the consequence is the same. There is an increased chance of cancer in the gastro-intestinal tract. We shall now examine why this is so, and look at the best way to combat it.

One of the more potent group of carcinogens, i.e. cancer producing agents, is the nitrosamines. They are substances known to be associated with increased incidence of cancers of the bladder, the oesophagus and the stomach. Sources of nitrosamines include cigarettes, chewing tobacco and snuff. Even non-smokers are exposed to them by way of sidestream smoke from cigarettes. Betel-nuts contain nitrosamines and as the nuts are chewed, the carcinogens are swallowed and enter the stomach and small intestine. Low levels of nitrosamines are present in cured meat products and malt beverages.

It is not only foods that provide us with nitrosamines. Cosmetics, corrosion inhibitors and a wide variety of rubber products have been found to contain ready-made nitrosamines. Even some rubber teats for baby bottles have been found to be contaminated with these substances.

Nitrosamines can also be formed in the stomach by the interaction of two other food constituents, namely, amines and nitrites. Nitrites are readily formed from nitrates, found, for example, in many vegetables and in drinking water and they are also added to cured meats, bacon, sausages and the like. Nitrites are excellent preservatives which is why they are added to foods.

Amines are natural constituents of foods (for example the characteristic smell of fish is due to them) but are also widely used in cosmetics and drugs. Neither amines nor nitrites are likely to cause cancer on their own but when they react together, the result is the carcinogenic nitrosamines. However, what has emerged from recent research is the fact that nitrosamines are more likely to be formed in a stomach that lacks hydrochloric acid. Once the nitrosamine has been formed it can then act anywhere within the digestive tract or be absorbed and produce its carcinogenic effect elsewhere.

Hence the simplest way to prevent nitrosamine formation is to inactivate the nitrites or the amines. The most effective agents for this are vitamins C and E which harmlessly detoxify nitrites. With these out of the way, there is no chance of nitrosamine formation. At the same time there is evidence appearing that vitamins C and E can also combine with and render harmless the preformed nitrosamines.

It would appear then that an adequate intake of vitamins C and E daily is the best protection against nitrosamimes but it is of even more importance if the stomach has ceased producing hydrochloric acid. For complete effectiveness these vitamins must be taken with food, preferably 100mg of each. If we wish to take hydrochloric acid by mouth what is the best way? It is possible to drink hydrochloric acid in a very diluted form but the practice is not recommended for self-treatment. It is likely to cause damage to the teeth, and heartburn. Usually it is introduced straight into the stomach via a tube so this is a technique reserved for the medical practitioner. There is also doubt as to the efficiency of hydrochloric acid administered in this way. A more useful supplement is to introduce hydrochloric acid in combined, solid form. Betaine hydrochloride is a white powder that can be produced in tablet form. Once dissolved this material yields 25 per cent of its weight as hydrochloric acid. The usual dose is between 60 and 500mg of betaine hydrochloride taken just after meals. Glutamic acid hydrochloride acts in a similar manner but in solution it yields only 20 per cent of its weight as hydrochloric acid. For this reason the recommended intake is 0.6 to 1.8g during meals.

There is no doubt that hydrochloric acid is an important secretory agent of the stomach but like so many other body constituents it is most effective when carefully controlled. Some people will go through life happily unaware of any deviation from the normal state of affairs. For those of the emotional type and who undergo periods of stress there must be an awareness of what excessive hydrochloric acid can do. It is more sensible for them to carry around nuts, dried fruit, protein wafers, malted milk tablets and the like, to counteract any hyperacidity, rather than alkali tablets. At the other end of the scale, once achlorhydria has been established, hydrochloric acid tablets and, more importantly, vitamins C and E should form part of their everyday supplementation.

5

Orthodox and Natural Treatments Examined

The main causes of acidity, dyspepsia, indigestion and stomach ulcer have already been discussed. People who suffer from these troubles in one of their various forms usually have a medical history which shows that they have long transgressed in more ways than one. Orthodox medical treatment for stomach ulcer usually consists of putting the patient on a 'soft, bland diet', supplemented with medicine. Failing that, surgical operation may be thought necessary.

In the light of advanced medical experience over the last twenty-five years, surgical operations for stomach ulcer are little short of folly, in many cases. Such operations merely attempt to cut off the effect. They make no attempt to remove the cause. Only in the extreme case, where the ulcer has eaten a hole through the stomach wall into the peritoneum, is surgical treatment warranted.

The soft, bland diet generally resorted to in hospitals is suppressive rather than curative. A soft, bland diet usually consists of milk and 'pappy' food. The ulcer is soothed rather than healed. No attempt is made to tell the patient where his diet was at fault. This is borne out by the fact that medical men generally fall victims to the usual catalogue of human ailments just like the people who, in desperation, go to them for advice! Often their diet is no different from that of the general run of the public.

After leaving hospital, ulcer sufferers, for want of better knowledge, invariably resume the very diet that caused the trouble, and generally suffer from the same trouble periodically throughout their lives, often ending in some incurable disease.

The Orthodox Theory of Causation

The orthodox concept does not admit that stomach ulcers are caused by a combination of faults in feeding. We have seen that the most likely cause of ulcers is an imbalance between the ulcer-producing factors like excess hydrochloric acid and digestive enzymes and the protective factors like mucus production, permeability of the lining and the rate at which cells of the lining are replaced. What causes this imbalance?

At one time it was thought that a 'focal infection' was the cause. This theory completely overlooked the fact that a focal infection itself (an abscessed tooth or tonsils) is merely a symptom of deep-seated ill-health and which, in turn, is most probably due to faulty nutrition.

The probability is that infection (from teeth, tonsils, or bowel) or defective blood-supply produces a local area of necrosis – the ulcer – and that the hydrochloric acid, which is always excessive in ulcer, keeps it open.

That was Dr Sippy's theory of ulcer-formation.

In the famous Sippy treatment, therefore, great dependence is put upon the use of alkalis such as bicarbonate of soda and milk of magnesia by mouth, in order to neutralize the excessive acid secretion.

The symptoms of ulcer in the stomach and duodenum are very characteristic. Dr Berkeley Moynihan used to emphasize this by saying that the patient in telling his story seems to be trying to recite the symptoms of ulcer as he remembers them' from having read them in a text-book on medicine.

Pain, or, rather, a sense of discomfort or rawness, referred to the pit of the stomach, coming on in the case of the stomach ulcer right after meals, in the case of the duodenal ulcer when the stomach is empty or just before meals, is the main symptom.

There are three serious complications. The commonest is haemorrhage, the patient vomiting a large amount of blood. The blood is dark and granular in appearance on account of its exposure to the gastric contents; it has been called coffee-ground vomitus.

Perforation,in which the ulcer eats its way through the stomach wall, allowing the stomach or duodenal contents to escape into the peritoneum, is of the utmost seriousness because of the peritonitis which follows. It demands immediate surgery. Fortunately its symptoms, such as pain, shock, and collapse, are so striking as to call attention to itself immediately and indicate the need of assistance.

The third complication is narrowing, or stenosis, of the pylorus (the outlet of the stomach), caused by the progressive contraction of the ulcer in healing. In treating the last condition, surgery is the most valued aid, the surgeon by the operation of gastro-enterostomy making a new outlet for the stomach at its lowest point.

The treatment of simple, uncomplicated ulcer is, besides the use of alkalis already mentioned, the institution of a diet. The diet should consist of food which has the highest combining power with hydrochloric acid and the lowest irritating power.

Milk, cream, and eggs are among such articles. Lean meat, mashed potatoes, well-cooked oatmeal, and cream soups also are well tolerated. Bread, unless it be toasted or stale, sweets, fried foods, heavy vegetables, and fruits in general are very irritating.

This summarizes the approach of the orthodox to the problem of stomach ulcer. The bland diet with hourly feedings of milk may help to relieve symptoms and may therefore be desirable during the first week of an active ulcer. There is no firm evidence, however, that a bland diet speeds healing or prevents recurrence.

A more practical approach is to eliminate foods that cause the patient distress such as fatty foods, spices, fruit juices and especially pepper. Coffee, tea, cocoa and cola all stimulate acid production and are taboo. Alcohol has the same effect. There is evidence that ulcers in those who do not smoke or who stop smoking heal more rapidly.

Remember that whilst food can neutralize acid, hence the advice to eat little and often, it also stimulates acid production. Diet of the above, orthodox type is not a completely effective way of neutralizing acid, so orthodox medicine looks further to medication with drugs or by surgery. Later we shall see how sensible dieting can both heal and prevent gastric ulceration.

Antacids

Although there is no proof that antacids promote healing or prevent occurrence of peptic ulcers, they are used in orthodox therapy to give only symptomatic relief. In general there are two types of antacids:

Absorbable antacids: Sodium bicarbonate, and calcium carbonate (chalk) are the most potent antacids but they are absorbed giving high levels of sodium and calcium minerals in the body. The result is a condition called alkalosis or milk-alkali syndrome. Symptoms include nausea, weakness and headache leading, after chronic ingestion, to kidney damage. Hence soluble antacids must be used with particular caution in those whose ulcer symptoms include vomiting and haemorrhage. Those who are dehydrated because of these conditions or who suffer from high blood-pressure or kidney trouble should not take absorbable antacids. Blood calcium levels may also rise leading to calcification in the soft tissues and organs of the body.

Non-absorbable antacids: Aluminium hydroxide is commonly used as an antacid and is regarded as relatively safe yet the following side-effects may occur. Phosphate depletion can result from the binding of phosphate by aluminium in the gastrointestinal tract. As a result, blood phosphate levels fall; the body then extracts more from the bone to make up the deficit so the bones weaken. The result is weakness, malaise and loss of appetite. Eventually the bone becomes so demineralized that breakages are relatively easy. Aluminium hydroxide may also cause constipation. Although alleged to be totally insoluble it is possible that some of the aluminium will dissolve and be absorbed. At high levels this mineral can be quite toxic.

Magnesia, which acts as magnesium hydroxide, is an effective antacid. It is often given with aluminium hydroxide to prevent the constipation induced by the latter. This is fine if the amount taken is carefully controlled but too much causes diarrhoea. As some magnesium is certainly absorbed, this treatment is not suitable for those suffering from kidney problems.

Bismuth salts were widely used in the past but are now falling into disrepute. This is largely due to lack of proof of their effectiveness, and their toxic effects which include loss of appetite, headache, malaise and skin reactions.

There is little to recommend any of the orthodox antacids in the treatment of peptic ulceration.

Anticholinergics

These drugs are given to delay emptying of the stomach which can be rapid in the case of uncomplicated duodenal ulcer. In this way antacid retention is prolonged and when taken in adequate doses, anticholinergics also diminish acid secretion. These drugs are most effective at night when regular hourly intake of antacids is impractical. Tincture of belladonna which is in this class of drugs is still widely used.

Like all drugs, however, anticholinergics provide their share of side-effects. Dry mouth, blurring of vision (or both), are not uncommon. Less common but more serious is urinary retention and glaucoma. Complete pyloric obstruction may develop in those with only partial obstruction. Anyone with oesophagitis or oesophageal ulcers cannot take anticholinergic drugs because of potential side-effects. For the same reason smokers should abstain whilst on these drugs.

Drugs that Reduce Acid Secretion

Many physicians now use therapeutic agents called histamine H_2 receptor blocking agents. These drugs act specifically by inhibiting the secretion of stomach acid. Usually the H_2 receptors in the stomach react to naturally-produced histamine by stimulating the production and secretion of hydrochloric acid. Hence by blocking these H_2 receptors in a specific manner, they no longer function and acid secretion stops.

Two such drugs are cimetidine and ranitidine. They are usually taken with each meal and at bedtime. Gastric acidity is lowered and healing of duodenal and gastric ulcers is promoted. Whilst symptoms are commonly relieved within the first week, complete healing of the ulcers may take between two and eight weeks. The usual length of treatment is four weeks. Not all ulcers are healed by these measures but the healing rate increases with length of treatment perhaps even up to 12 weeks. Unfortunately, the longer the therapy lasts the more chances there are of side-effects.

What are the likely side-effects? Diarrhoea, muscle

pain, dizziness and skin rash may occasionally occur. These are relatively mild side-effects but there are more serious ones. Impotence, lack of sperms in semen and other effects induced by the anti-sex hormone properties of cimetidine have been reported although rarely. In addition cases of acute pancreatitis and nephritis (inflammation of the kidneys) have been associated with cimetidine.

Ranitidine allegedly causes less side-effects than cimetidine but this may simply reflect its less widespread use. The chances are that as more patients are treated with ranitidine, side-effects will begin to appear.

Having established that H_2 antagonists will heal peptic ulcers in most patients, the question remains on how to prevent their recurrence. When treatment with these drugs is stopped after ulcer healing, up to eighty per cent of patients will have ulcer recurrence within one year. For this reason, the patient is often put onto maintenance therapy at a lower dose. Despite this, experience in the United Kingdom has indicated a remission rate of thirty per cent in the case of duodenal ulcers and that of twenty per cent in gastric ulcers in the first twelve months of maintenance therapy. There are however unexplained differences between patients in various countries. In duodenal ulcers recurrence during one year maintenance on ranitidine was twenty-six per cent in the UK; sixteen per cent in West Germany and a massive sixty per cent in Austria and Belgium.

There are no obvious reasons for these variations.

Age, sex, smoking habits and drug tolerance appeared to play no part. What was apparent, however, was that when maintenance therapy discontinued after one year, relapses occurred at the same rate as before treatment. The conclusion reached was that drug therapy with H_2 receptor antagonists merely suppresses the disease and does not alter its natural history.

In 1982 a World Congress of Gastroenterology, held in Stockholm, assessed the efficiency of these drugs. Whilst there was no doubt of their usefulness in healing ulcers no clear-cut decision was reached on how to prevent their recurrence in chronic disease. The choice lay between long-term maintenance therapy, with the risk of side-effects, and surgery.

One speaker suggested there were signs that the natural history of gastric and duodenal ulcers in the UK was changing to a 'less aggressive' form. Fewer patients were being presented for emergency surgery because of perforation or haemorrhage. This trend had actually started before the H_2 antagonist drugs had been introduced so there was some other, less obvious reason.

Unhappily though, it was reported that the total incidence of ulcer disease is not falling and the sad conclusion was that more and more patients would end up on long-term drug therapy. No one suggested that dietary principles could be the best cure and prevention of peptic ulcers.

One of the more serious controversies concerning cimetidine therapy was centred on the possibility of the drug causing gastric cancer. Out of 9,504 patients who had taken cimetidine, gastric cancer was diagnosed in 74. Twenty-three were diagnosed before treatment had started; 29 had gastric cancer within six months of starting therapy. Only 8 patients out of 8,994 controls (who did not receive the drug) developed gastric cancer over the same period of one year. It is possible that cimetidine had been used unwittingly to treat gastric cancer (which had been there all the time) according to those reporting the trials. It was obvious however that a possible association between cimetidine and gastric cancer had not been disproved, according to one researcher.

Liquorice
Liquorice has a soothing (or demulcent) action on the mucous membranes which is why it is used to relieve coughs and sore throats. It also has an expectorant action which helps to remove the phlegm that is often the cause of throat irritation. This demulcent property is the reason why liquorice is also a traditional remedy for peptic ulceration.

Liquorice has mild anti-inflammatory properties but in addition it can also act like the corticosteroid hormones produced in the adrenal glands. The latter are undesirable so the ideal preparation of liquorice for treating ulcers would be one that retained the demulcent and anti-inflammatory properties but reduced the hormone-like activity. Such a preparation is deglycyrrhizinised liquorice and it has found great use in healing peptic ulcers.

Another approach is to modify chemically a constituent of liquorice to produce an anti-ulcer drug. This is called carbenoxolone. Like all liquorice preparations it functions by reducing the inflammation around the ulcer and by causing the secretion of large amounts of thick protective mucus that cover the ulcer. Hence by preventing contact of hydrochloric acid with the ulcer, the mucus allows natural healing to take place. At the same time liquorice preparations stimulate cell regeneration which accelerates the rate of healing.

Because liquorice and its derivatives still retain adrenal cortex hormone-like activities, they can still exert an effect upon the minerals of the body. This leads to sodium and water retention, causing oedema. At the same time there is excessive loss of potassium in the urine along with excessive alkaline conditions in the body. High blood-pressure has been reported as well as a mild, reversible, diabetic-like condition. Heartburn can follow the ingestion of carbenoxolone in tablet form.

Liquorice and its constituents can therefore be regarded as natural agents in the successful treatment of gastric and duodenal ulcers but their use must be tempered with caution. In moderate amounts, the root can have a positive beneficial effect but at the same time its possible side-effects must be monitored since they can be detrimental. Deglycyrrhizinised liquorice appears to be the preparation of choice in terms of safety and efficacy.

Vitamin A and Gastric Ulcers
Although treatment of gastric ulcers with vitamin A can hardly be regarded as orthodox since relatively high doses are required, there is increasing interest

in using this natural food constituent as a therapeutic agent. It is well known that vitamin A has a
protective action on skin and mucous membranes;
indeed it is one of its accepted, essential functions.
For this reason it was reasoned that the vitamin
had the potential for exerting a similar action
against gastric ulcer. This hypothesis has been
tested in a multi-centre, randomized, controlled
trial of vitamin A in sixty patients with chronic
gastric ulcers. The trial took place in Hungary and
was reported in *The Lancet* towards the end of
1982.

There were three groups of patients. One group
was treated only with antacids; the second group
received similar antacids with the addition of
150,000IU of vitamin A daily; the third group were
given the same doses of vitamin A and antacids
daily with the addition of cyproheptadine, an
antihistamine drug, also daily. All patients were
treated for four weeks. Ulcer sizes were measured
before and after treatment in each case.

All ulcers were reduced to a significant degree
but those patients receiving vitamin A experienced
a significantly greater reduction in size than those
treated just with antacids. The authors concluded
that 'a beneficial effect of vitamin A has been
indicated in the prevention and treatment of stress
ulcers in patients'.

No simple clinical trial is accepted by the medical
fraternity as conclusive until it has been repeated
with similar success. The above trial was conducted
on patients with stress-induced gastric ulcers. It
was therefore repeated on patients suffering from

chronic and recurrent gastric ulcers and reported in the *International Journal of Tissue Reactions* in 1983. The second trial was a randomized, prospective study of sixty patients with chronic gastric ulcer. One group received antacids only; the second group were given antacids plus 50,000IU vitamin A three times daily and the third group received the same medication as the second group but with the addition of an antihistamine drug. As before, treatment was continued for four weeks. The number of patients with completely healed ulcers was higher in the groups which received vitamin A. In addition, the reduction in ulcer size was greater in patients who were given vitamin A. The authors concluded that 'vitamin A has a beneficial effect in the process of ulcer healing in patients with chronic gastric ulcer'.

One pleasing aspect of both trials was the complete lack of toxic side-effects despite the relatively high intakes of vitamin A. They suggest that 150,000IU daily for four weeks is a dose of the vitamin easily tolerated over this period. The excellent response is an indication of natural treatment. On the other hand, as we shall see later, these results also suggest that prevention of gastric ulceration can be brought about by an adequate intake of this vitamin throughout life.

Gastric ulcers can be thought of as a pre-cancerous state and significant negative correlation has been reported between body levels of vitamin A and the development of various cancers. In other words low levels of the vitamin appear to be found regularly in cases of cancer of the lung, bladder and skin. The results of these two trials indicate a possible role for gastric protection in the prevention of the development of gastric cancer from gastric ulcer.

The Use of Cabbage Juice

Professor Garnet Cheney, of the Stanford Medical School, California, has had success with cabbage juice in the treatment of stomach ulcers. He says that it is the Vitamin C factor in the juice which has such powerful healing qualities. This may only be partly true since the same researcher reported a unique factor, called vitamin U, in cabbage leaves and other vegetables. This has been called the anti-ulcer vitamin. Vitamin U has been isolated from cabbage leaves and has also been produced by chemical synthesis. It is known under the trade names of *Caboagin-U, Epadyn-U, Vitas U* and *Ardesyl*.

Cabbage juice is quite a pleasant drink, but the processing really requires an electric juicer, and these are expensive. It would be wise to regard cabbage juice as a supplementary factor in the cure of stomach ulcer, and not to place the onus of cure upon it. Whatever the virtues of cabbage juice, it is not a substitute for the curative and preventative principles set out in this book. Most cabbages are raised on soils fertilized with chemical manures and this reduces their vitamin content and nutritional value.

Garlic

Oil of garlic has remarkable healing properties and

has been used in Europe and Asia for centuries. Garlic is a cleanser and kills the unfriendly bacteria *B. coli* in the large intestine, thereby lightening the duties of the liver and spleen. Garlic improves the appetite, reduces blood tension and helps to prevent thrombosis. It is excellent in respiratory troubles; is highly regarded as a nerve tonic and remedies flatulence and diarrhoea. It is recognized as a most valuable intestinal antiseptic. Garlic capsules, each containing three minims of pure oil of garlic, are readily available.

Herbal Remedies

We have discussed already one herbal remedy for peptic ulcers, that is, liquorice. In addition, however, there are other traditional remedies for gastric conditions and one of the better established and more effective ones is althaea root, otherwise known as marshmallow root. Its main active constituent is mucilage but it also contains sterols, asparagin and lecithin, all of which contribute to its beneficial effect. Marshmallow has a demulcent action combined with an emollient or softening and soothing effect. For this reason the root is recommended for gastritis and enteritis but its specific indications are gastric and duodenal ulcers. The usual dose is between 2 and 5g of the dried root three times daily. A more effective preparation is a combination of marshmallow with symphytum.

Symphytum: This is more commonly known as comfrey and it is active in either the root or leafy form. Both have a demulcent action that is due to their content of mucilage, allantoin, symphitine and echimidine. They have found use in the treatment of gastric and duodenal ulcers. The usual dose of dried root or dried leaves is 2-4g or 4-8g respectively, taken at the rate of three doses per day.

Slippery Elm Bark: Also known as ulmus, it is another rich source of mucilage which explains its beneficial actions as a demulcent and emollient. Unlike most herbal remedies it contains significant amounts of starch which contributes to its food properties. Specifically it is used to help heal gastric and duodenal ulcers. The powdered bark is usually extracted with water at the rate of 1 part bark to 8 parts water. The liquid (4-16cc) is drunk three times daily. There are however many commercial preparations of dried bark extract that are more convenient to take.

Failure of Ulcer Operations

With the exception of urgent surgical operations to repair the damage where an ulcer has eaten a hole right through to the peritoneum, ulcer operations have a record of failure. To cut out an ulcer and draw the wall of the stomach together, cannot possibly be described as a 'cure'. But it can be described as a very dangerous intrusion into an area of the body that Nature, in her wisdom, has carefully and hermetically sealed, and is often followed by serious results for the patient. If the patient recovers and goes on in the same old dietetic way, further ulcers will occur, and what then? More operations?

Dr Richard Harrison (USA) expressed this view: 'A man or woman who has stomach ulcer is sick all over. It is utterly ridiculous and dangerous to treat a stomach ulcer by localised medication or by surgical removal.'

Dr Walter C. Alvarez, of the Mayo Clinic, said: 'If the patient is worrisome and temperamental, operation is probably useless.'

What pain-racked, nerve-racked ulcer sufferer is *not* worrisome and temperamental? By this time he is beside himself with suffering. Dr James Brown, in a treatise on the subject, points out that even after an operation, 'treatment of the complaint has only begun'.

In his book *Peptic Ulcer*, Dr T. L. Cleave states that every year 30,000 human stomachs are removed in operating theatres in the United Kingdom. After praising the skill of the surgeons, Dr Cleave points out that the operation carries liabilities. There is loss of energy and the patient may be compared to 'a bird that has lost a handful of feathers from one wing'. Another liability never usually mentioned, says Dr Cleave, is that the original cause of the trouble continues to operate and 'other diseases may supervene in the future'.

Diet Supersedes Surgery
Dr B. P. Allinson, a member of the Royal College of Surgeons, in the course of a lecture given in London on unnecessary operative surgery said:

The question arises as to how much abdominal

surgery is justified, and here again I personally am no doubt apt to form any conclusions from the failures I have seen, though, speaking in general, I think that most surgery that is performed for ulcers should not be performed. There is much surgery for ulceration, and I see a great many of the failures of this surgery, more especially of what are called short-circuit operations. In these cases one has to deal with an additional disability in the form of the operative interference that has taken place.

I think that adequate natural methods, principally dietetic methods, can deal with digestive ulceration, especially with chronic digestive ulceration, much more satisfactorily than surgery can, and in this case I would especially emphasise the non-toxic diet, that is, avoiding all poisons, especially tea, coffee, tobacco, alcohol, and all flesh foods.

On a diet of that description not only do these ulcers heal but they remain healed which is important, because one of the surgeon's dicta in the subject is: 'Oh, it is all very well; you may heal an ulcer with a diet, but it will come back again, and then an emergency will arise'.

That again, as I say, is true within the surgeon's own experience, but I have dealt with quite a large number of ulcers, principally duodenal ulcers, which are more common than gastric ulcers, and they have healed and they have remained healed.

I have had two relapses out of a number, but even in those cases the ulcers healed again after the relapse and remained healed. If the surgeon were to know that a proper diet would heal the ulcers perfectly, as long as the individual adhered to it, then perhaps he would modify his view about the necessity of surgery.

It is important to remember also the consequences

of partial or total removal of the stomach by surgery. The operation results in loss of hydrochloric acid production; loss of stomach digestive enzymes; loss of intrinisic factor secretion. The latter, as we have seen, will prevent the absorption of vitamin B_{12}, so pernicious anaemia may result. This is why regular injections of vitamin B_{12} are essential to anyone who has had a partial or complete gastrectomy. The consequences of lack of hydrochloric acid production have already been discussed.

Surgery's Attack on the Ulcer

A development in operative surgery for ulcers is to sever the vagus nerve. This is called vagotomy. The theory behind this new and desperate exploration into the abdominal cavity is as follows. Some ulcer cases are nervy, worrisome, restless types. While they are in this state, the gastric juice is constantly flowing, due to the fact that the vagus nerve connects the stomach with the brain. If the stomach could be disconnected from the brain, by cutting the vagus nerve, then the stomach would not be affected by the state of the patient's brain, and his worries, etc.

That is the theory of the surgery, but it is not now a common approach in Britain and the USA to attack the problem of stomach ulcers by severing the vagus nerve. The more advanced medical man, who puts his faith in sound nutrition, views this surgical intrusion into the human body with alarm. He points out that the vagus nerve not only connects the stomach to the brain, but supplies branches to the heart, lungs, throat and abdomen.

To sever this vitally important nerve may have serious repercussions on the sympathetic nervous system which controls these organs. It is a clumsy, even dangerous method of attempting to control overactivity on the part of the nervous system and the flow of gastric fluids. It is significant that the usual sensational claims of success have not been made in the case of this type of operation.

Where Orthodox Treatment Fails

Orthodox medical treatment is notorious for its failure to cure ulcers in the digestive tract because:

1. It makes no attempt to correct the dietetic errors of the patient.

2. It resorts to a 'soft, bland diet' which, while temporarily coating the ulcer, is in its nature constipating and deficient in vitamins and minerals. Indeed, fresh fruits and raw salad vegetables are not permitted because they might 'irritate' the ulcer! Orthodox medicine quite overlooks the fact that these sores can only be healed by raising the purity and tone of the blood-stream, and by maintaining this purity and tone permanently. It was the absence of vitamins and minerals that largely caused the ulcer in the first place. No ulcer is likely to form in the digestive tract of a person whose blood-stream had been consistently fed on foods rich in vitamins and minerals.

3. To resort to antacid powders, bicarbonate of soda and milk of magnesia to supply alkalines is just another example of the educated ignorance so

common in orthodox medical practice.

4. Surgery is rarely necessary for the narrowing of the pylorus caused by an ulcer. This condition rarely fails to respond to a diet of well-diluted fruit juices or vegetable juices, which have an alkaline reaction in the body.

6

Views on Causes and Cures

Orthodox medical men put far too much emphasis on worry and the strains of modern life as the main causes of ulcers. Nevertheless doctors do get the impression that peptic ulcers are commonest in tense, anxious people. Nervous tension makes them worse so sufferers are advised to calm themselves down if they can. What is certain is that smoking, even though it may help calm some people, will make peptic ulcers worse.

Sir Robert McCarrison, who was for some years medical officer among the Hunza in Northern India, failed to find one case of stomach ulcer, kidney disease or heart disease among those people over a period of nine years. The Hunza live on vegetables, cheese, fruit, milk and coarse grain mostly, with meat as a luxury once in a while. These people also live calm unstressful lives without the problems and pace of modern civilization and this too may be a factor, along with that of their diet, in keeping them free of the scourge of peptic ulcers.

Women and Children Now Ulcer Victims
The following excerpts from a cable from New

York, published in the press of 29 January 1961, are of interest:

'Stomach ulcers, once considered an exclusively male disease, are now attacking women and children in alarming numbers. U.S. research figures this week showed that the number of women sufferers had risen by about 350 per cent in the past 20 years. A British doctor found that nine of a family of 13 had duodenal ulcers. Doctors were fast revising old theories about what foods an ulcer sufferer should eat or avoid.

'American doctors are staging an all-out attack on the ailment that in the U.S. alone costs the nation £222 million a year in medical bills and loss of work time. Authorities point out that there is a growing number of female ulcer sufferers due to the increased commitments of the working woman. "Today's woman is competing actively with man outside her home, while inside she has become a full partner in marriage, sharing the decisions that affect her family's future," a noted psychiatrist said this week . . .

'In a recent British project, doctors discovered that . . . dieting with bland foods does not increase the rate of healing of peptic ulcers . . .'

At the Mayo Clinic in Rochester, Minnesota, 2,000 patients being treated for arthritis with aspirin-type medications were found to have four times as many ulcers as the other patients. Other doctors have observed that large amounts of aspirin taken by ulcer sufferers coincide with bleeding.

'A British study found more ulcers among truck drivers and baggage clerks than among professional men. On the lowest social level of unskilled labourers, the men's ulcer rate was found to be 116 per cent of the national average. On the highest, the rate was only 48 per cent.'

An Ulcer Specialist Supports Our Views

Fortunately, there is a growing, if small, percentage of medical practitioners who are leading the profession in the new and sounder approach to the problem of acidity and stomach ulcer.

One of these is the famous Scottish doctor, Dr Fyfe Robertson, who was himself a sufferer from stomach ulcer for years. He is a recognized authority on the subject and has cured hundreds of very bad cases, including himself. Dr Fyfe Robertson has no hesitation in saying that it is the 'degradation of food' during the past century that has given rise to the alarming increase in stomach ulcer. He explains that the degradation of food has been due to '"Scientific" farming, which alters the nature of things that grow in the soil—by the use of artificial fertilisers and sprays to kill plant diseases and pests; and injections to fight animal diseases. Food-processing methods which rob foods of most of their virtue—in the case of white flour, of almost everything except starch. Use of preservatives, "improvers", colouring and flavouring agents, of artificial chemical substances which are often poisonous. Loss of nutritive value through increasing staleness of foods. In spite of better transport, many foodstuffs are older and staler when they reach the consumer than they were 50 years ago.

'And freezing, gas storage, chemical preserving

have advantages—but they do not improve foods. The nostalgia of the elderly for the foods of their youth is justified; they were fresher, tastier and more wholesome, because they were whole foods.

'Apologists for modern food practices excuse them individually because their effects, individually, are so small. But cumulatively they are enormous.'

The Menace of Preservative Poisons

Dr Robertson continues: 'Consider a diet including dyed, frozen, gassed, canned, chemically preserved and flavoured foods; eggs from hens unnaturally fed and kept; stale fish; stale vegetables often grown by suspect methods; processed cheese instead of original real cheese; "full fruit" jam preserved with sulphur dioxide and chemically dyed; white sugar, vitaminless and consumed in over-large quantities; cereal foods heat-treated before the consumer gets them. "A man is what he eats", so the old saying goes. Would you rule out the possibility that these things, operating daily for years and in the unborn child, may be the cause of bodily changes and damage? We have largely abolished the dirt disease, but the most significant medical fact today is the alarming increase in chronic degenerative diseases. Now these degenerative diseases are rarely found among people, primitive or civilized, who eat fresh, whole, unprocessed, naturally grown foods. The kind of food changes outlined here have taken place in most industrialised countries at about the same time with the rise in ulcers, particularly duodenal.'

What One Experiment Proved

'Brilliant physician Sir Robert McCarrison, one of the greatest figures in the science of nutrition, proved that differences in the physique and disease incidence among India's people could be directly related to food differences.

'Feeding rats from the same stock for 700 days (equal to 50 human years) on three human diets selected from different areas, he found that those given the worst in protein, vitamins, minerals, and over-rich in starch suffered most in health. Of the rats worst fed 29 per cent had duodenal and gastric ulcers. Those fed on a 'natural' balanced diet had no ulcers.

'When in another experiment McCarrison fed one group on the best diet and another on one of the kinds of foods eaten by the British poor, he had to segregate the "British" rats to stop them eating each other. Post-mortems of all rats after 190 days (equal to 16 human years) showed gastric ulcers, gastritis, enteritis, colitis in the "British" group, but none in the properly fed group. Even the psychiatrist must concede the significance of results like these. And the ulcer victim, drinking his alkalis, anxiously eating his miserable diet, coping with nausea, hiding the pain that grips and gnaws, fearing the meal his hunger pain makes so desirable, may wonder why findings so convincing as McCarrison's have not led to a new approach to this problem. Basically orthodox medical treatment has not changed in many years. There have, of course, been fashions—many.'

Old Treatment Still Used

Dr Robertson continues: 'Sippy's milk and alkali diet, introduced in 1915, still holds the field, with refinements, with orthodox medical men. This is based on the belief that ulcers are caused by the stomach's hydrochloric acid—that the patient's own digestive juice is digesting the protein of his stomach wall, which is probably true, but as the "last link" of the chain-causes. The aim therefore is to absorb it with chemical absorbents, to use it up with frequent meals.

'Since it is believed that the high stomach activity often found in ulcer cases aggravates damage and pain, drugs to reduce muscular activity are also given. The diet mainstay is milk, with eggs second, and the drill is frequent meals. Some doctors give foods or alkalis or both every two hours. The latest fad is the sucking all day of alkali-loaded milk tablets, since alkalis (owing to stomach emptying) do not act for more than about 15 minutes.

'No roughage is allowed—not even the tiniest, as it is believed that pain is caused by food passing over the ulcer. If the diet is bland, it is also unappetising and dreary. The prohibitions are immense, quite often unnecessary and psychologically disastrous. Surgical treatment has had many fashions, the tendency being to more and more drastic methods. A new technique, severance of the nerves controlling stomach movement and acid secretion, is already discredited. Surgery has improved and for some conditions it is essential, but it is not now so lightly recommended.'

Stomach Ulcers—A Deficiency Ailment

Dr D. T. Quigley in *The National Malnutrition* wrote: 'The first treatment for stomach ulcer which attained any great attention by the medical profession was the so-called Sippy treatment. This treatment consisted in neutralizing the highly acid condition of the stomach with chalk and other alkalines, but it also included hourly feedings of milk or cream and orange juice. Sippy knew nothing whatever of vitamins, and perhaps never thought of such a thing as mineral deficiency in this class of disease, but through a fortuitous accident his treatment provided the patient with calcium and also with the vitamins contained in butter fat, milk, and orange juice.

'This treatment supplies only a part of the whole deficiency needs of a person with this type of disease, but it was so great an improvement over the deficiency diets which produced the disease that many patients were temporarily cured. Sippy and the others of his time did not recognize the fact that the patient needed not a temporary treatment, but a permanent one. They did not recognize the fact that the ulcers were due to dietary deficiences and that the patients must be put on a correct diet for the rest of their lives. They assumed that the patient was consuming a normal diet, and that the ulcer was due to some mysterious and unexplainable happening which in some way was connected with the production of too much acid in the stomach. We now know that the acid is the defence mechanism. It is the only mechanism the stomach has for fighting back against irritations from without. The person suffering with this kind of disease always has some degree of scurvy. The scurvy has produced bad teeth and infected gums. The bad teeth and infected gums have caused pus to be swallowed into the stomach, sometimes at the rate of about a teaspoonful every hour. The swallowing of pus produces local irritation. The irritation calls out the increased stomach secretion. Continuation of the irritation results in an increase of hydrochloric acid, leading eventually to ulceration. These happenings cover a period of years, and by the time the ulcer appears in the stomach or duodenum the whole gastro-intestinal tract is diseased and along with it the liver duct and gall bladder. The ulcer is a focal breakdown in a completely diseased gastro-intestinal canal.

'On the clinical side, many internists and some surgeons have come to consider vitamin C as a cure for stomach ulcers. Here they are recognizing a truth, but only a part of the whole truth—lack of vitamin C is undoubtedly one of the predominant causes of stomach ulcer. A complete treatment would mean a treatment with all other vitamins and minerals lacking in the individual's diet, as well as with vitamin C.'

Gayelord Hauser on the Cure of Stomach Ulcer
Gayelord Hauser, American nutritional scientist, confirmed most of the conclusions arrived at in this book when he wrote in *Diet Does It!*:

'In few instances has the diet used in the correction of disease been so disgracefully inadequate as that given to persons suffering from ulcers of the stomach or duodenum. The Sippy diet, which consists of taking milk and cream every two hours, was first used when the science of nutrition was unknown. Yet it is still in general use. The principles upon which it was built, however, are as unsound today as they were then. An ulcer is nothing more than a sore in the wall of the stomach or intestine. The normal stomach secretes strong hydrochloric acid from which the stomach and intestinal walls are usually protected by a covering of thick mucus. The ulcerated spot, however, cannot produce mucus by which to protect itself; yet the ulcer cannot heal readily with strong acid pouring over it.'

'The reason for recommending that an ulcer patient drink milk and cream every two hours is that milk combines with hydrochloric acid and cream inhibits its flow; thus acid is kept from the ulcer until it has a chance to heal. The person who wishes to recover from an ulcer should drink a glass of milk every two hours or, if the pain is severe, half a glass every hour. If the patient is overweight, skim milk can be used. The difficulty with a milk diet, however, is that it is inadequate in almost all vitamins and in iron and copper. Cases have been reported in the *Journal of the American Medical Association* of people who have developed both scurvy and beriberi, diseases caused by an almost total lack of vitamin C and B, while living on a milk diet. The milk and cream diet, therefore, must be modified in order to make it adequate, to increase rapid healing, and to prevent the recurrence of ulcers.

Hauser on Vitamins for Ulcer

'Two new methods used in the correction of ulcer have met with marked success. One is the giving of massive doses of vitamin A, which maintains the health of mucous membrane lining the walls of the stomach and intestine. The other treatment is that of giving 1,000 milligrams of vitamin C daily for three days in the form of 100 milligram tablets; the amount is increased by 100 milligrams daily until the dosage reaches 2,000 milligrams; this amount should then be continued indefinitely. This large amount of Vitamin C stimulates the formation of scar tissue and causes the ulcer to heal rapidly. Citrus juices are usually avoided because of the citric acid they contain, but vegetable juices, especially carrot juice, can be used freely. (Citrus juices can, however, be used if well diluted with water.) These two methods are excellent and are to be recommended to anyone with an active ulcer. Even with whole milk and ample amounts of vitamins A and C, the diet is still markedly inadequate. The person with an ulcer must obtain the vitamins of the B family. At least a half cup of short-cooked wheatgerm should be eaten each morning, and a tablespoonful of powdered brewer's yeast stirred into milk should be taken after each meal. All liquids should be drunk through a straw. (This is to avoid swallowing air which may result in flatulence.) Iron and copper can be obtained from a serving of wheatgerm.'

The Bioflavonoids and Stomach Ulcers

Recent research indicates that improved healing

follows when vitamin C is taken in conjunction with the bioflavonoid complex. A special tablet is available which contains 100mg of the bioflavonoid complex, 95mg vitamin C and 5mg rose hips. These tablets can be taken for stomach ulcers as well as, or in replacement of vitamin C tablets. We suggest that a bioflavonoid and vitamin C tablet be taken twice daily, after meals, in addition to the vitamin C tablets already listed.

'When Cured, Keep On Vital Diet', said Hauser
'Fruit and vegetables need be puréed only if they are not well tolerated otherwise. Thorough chewing is essential. After the ulcer has healed it is of extreme importance to continue the Vital Diet indefinitely to maintain healthy scar tissue. Otherwise an ulcer will quickly recur. I believe it is correct to say that if a Vital Diet is maintained, day after day and year after year, infections and the many resulting handicaps will be a thing of the past.'

Thirteen Curative Principles

Having dealt earlier in this book with the causes of indigestion and stomach ulcer, the curative principles will naturally consist of not doing those very things which singly, or together, caused the trouble. The first principle of curing any ailment is to stop causing it. To put the matter more positively, we have summarized the advice given by the world's leading medical scientists in regard to the cure of indigestion, ulcers, and stomach troubles generally into thirteen simple principles, which any sufferer can understand and apply:

Eat Less
(1) Eat much less than you were in the habit of eating. Eat simply. Make a meal of one course—one kind of mild fruit, or salad, or lightly cooked vegetables. (Study the Science of Life book *Eating for Health*).

Take Supplements
(2) Build up your starved nervous organization by systematically taking the B_1, B complex and calcium tablets recommended in the diet for stomach ulcers.

Protein and Ulcers: Experiments with laboratory animals have disclosed that if they are kept on a diet deficient in protein, one hundred per cent of them develop ulcers of the duodenum or stomach. Similarly, persons with stomach or duodenal ulcers are often found to have lived on diets lacking in protein. Even when stomach ulcers in such persons have healed, they soon recur if too little protein is included in the daily diet. Having developed a stomach ulcer, it cannot be healed quickly, however, merely by increasing one's daily intake of protein. Why? Because all protein foods stimulate the flow of the gastric juices, which contain a powerful acid (hydrochloric) needed to digest proteins. This acid erodes and irritates the raw surface of the stomach ulcer, giving rise to pain. The first thing to be done therefore is to help nature to establish a protective coating over the ulcer and thereby expedite the healing process. To do this it is necessary to cut down one's intake of protein foods to a minimum for several weeks. This gives the ulcerous surface a respite from the irritation set up by the acid mentioned. No more than two or three ounces of cheese should be taken daily during this period. It is best to omit meat altogether for the first two weeks, as meat is inferior to cheese in nutritional qualities and is not so easily digested. Wheatgerm can be used later and may be short cooked if desired.

Cheese: Cheese, as we have seen, is a more valuable form of protein than meat and has more energy value and nourishment. In addition, cheese contains lactic acid which aids digestion and is rich in calcium, essential to strong nerves and healthy tissue. Packeted cheese is generally processed and it is therefore advisable to purchase unprocessed block cheese.

Take Alkaline-forming Foods

(3) See that approximately 80 per cent of your food consists of alkaline-forming foods (fruit, raw salad vegetables, cooked vegetables, milk and dried fruits) and only 20 per cent of the acid-forming foods (meat, fish, eggs, cheese, bread, concentrated starches and sugary foods). Not alkaline powders but alkaline foods and diluted fruit juices possess the secret of neutralizing excessive acidity in the stomach, and maintaining the proper acid/alkaline balance in the blood. That is a simple, easy-to-remember principle of first-class health.

Avoid Incompatible Feeding

(4) Avoid incompatible feeding in the following ways:

(a) Don't eat a protein and a concentrated starch or sugary food at the same meal;

(b) Don't eat a concentrated starch food (such as white bread and potatoes) and an acid fruit at the same meal;

(c) Don't eat a milk pudding or drink milk on top of a meat meal;

(d) Don't eat raw and cooked vegetables or raw and stewed fruits at the same meal.

In the case of (a), (b), and (c) protein foods require

an acid solution for their digestion. They are primarily digested by the gastric juice secreted in the stomach. All other foods require an alkaline solution for their digestion. This is secreted in the mouth and is mixed with the food in the saliva. A sick stomach cannot be both acid and alkaline at the same time. This is a difficult enough feat for a healthy stomach to achieve.

Make Good Vitamin Deficiencies

(5) All vitamin and mineral deficiencies must be made good and maintained as a regular routine of life. The following vitamins, which are the great healing agents for stomach ulcers, and also ulcers of the duodenum and pylorus, should be taken consistently before each meal, three times daily. They can all be taken together.

1 Vitamin E tablet or capsule (100mg)
1 Vitamin A tablet or capsules (2,500 IU*)
1 Vitamin B₁ tablet (10mg)
1 Vitamin B complex tablet (10mg strength)
1 Vitamin C tablet (250mg)
2 calcium tablets, white (75mg each of calcium)
*(If vitamin A capsules are used instead of tablets, these should be taken after meals.)

Once daily, a pantothenic acid tablet should be taken (at least 100mg). Where the diet is rich in calcium foods—milk, cream, cheese—the calcium tablets may be omitted. Such a diet would include 2 pints (1.1 litres) of milk and 4oz (115g) of cheese daily.

Extra B vitamins are needed for a variety of

reasons. Persistent use of antacids, for example, particularly amongst older people can lead to impaired absorption of vitamin B_1 with subsequent low body levels of the vitamin. It is important therefore to take vitamin B_1 supplements to ensure an adequate intake. Younger people are not immune either as they too can suffer from persistent dyspepsia. One consequence of too little vitamin B_1 is constipation so taking supplements of the vitamin whilst suffering from one gastro-intestinal complaint can prevent another.

Vitamin B_2 is needed to maintain healthy mucous membranes and it can have a preventative and curative effect on those suffering from mouth ulcers. There is no doubt that sometimes the type of person likely to suffer from peptic ulcers is also the type to develop mouth ulcers. Hence it is sound supplementation to ensure an adequate daily intake of vitamin B_2, also in those liable to gastric and duodenal ulcers.

When nicotinamide, or vitamin B_3, is deficient, one of the common symptoms is gastro-intestinal upsets characterized by nausea, vomiting and sometimes inflammation of the mouth and digestive tract. These symptoms, as we have seen, are also associated with gastric and duodenal ulceration so a daily supplement of nicotinamide is a useful insurance policy.

Pantothenic acid is a B vitamin that is needed in the production of anti-stress hormones. Hence if the individual is the stressed, nervous or overwrought type, the result can be an increased tendency for them to develop gastric or duodenal ulcers. Adequate pantothenic acid and, indeed, vitamin C, also will at least ensure that anti-stress hormone production is not deficient and the tendency to produce ulcers is lessened.

Need for Fat

When insufficient fat is included in the diet, foods leave the stomach fairly rapidly and the walls of the stomach are then exposed to the action of strong hydrochloric acid for lengthy periods. We advise that a little fatty food be eaten at every meal and after meals, a teaspoonful of olive oil be taken.

Vitamin A

Quite apart from the value of vitamin A in building a healthy lining to the stomach, intestines, throat and lungs, it is vitally important for resistance to all infections. In addition though, as we have seen, high doses of this vitamin can actually heal ulcers. It is therefore quite possible that adequate intakes daily may help prevent ulceration in the first place.

How Vitamin C Heals Ulcers

Vitamin C strengthens connective tissue and the walls of the blood vessels, both of which are essential in the healing of stomach ulcers. Dr John Marks of Downing College, Cambridge, England has written in his *Guide to the Vitamins* that in gastro-intestinal disturbances vitamin C deficiency may arise through impaired absorption. The beneficial effect of vitamin C upon wound healing makes it essential that adequate amounts be administered in all cases of gastric and duodenal ulcers especially as 'ulcer diets' are usually deficient in the vitamin.

Some advanced doctors in the USA are getting remarkably good results with 1500 milligrams of vitamin C daily. However, the important thing to do is to heal the ulcer as quickly as possible. The quantity mentioned—1500 milligrams of vitamin C daily—is obtained by taking six 250 milligram vitamin C tablets daily.

What Vitamin E Does

Animal experiments have indicated that when subjected to stress, those given large amounts of vitamin E developed far fewer and less serious ulcers than those who received nothing but a standard diet. For example, in one experiment reported in the *American Journal of Clinical Nutrition* in 1972, Dr G. F. Solomon and his colleagues compared rats that were subjected to stressful conditions. One group received 50mg vitamin E orally twice a day along with one meal; the other group received just the one meal. After 12 days, the unsupplemented rats developed 78 per cent more ulceration than those receiving vitamin E.

It is possible that vitamin E can have a sparing effect in vitamin A deficiency. As long ago as 1946, Dr J. L. Jensen published in the journal *Science* his finding that vitamin E prevented stomach ulcers in rats receiving very low amounts of vitamin A. Later, a follow-up experiment was reported by Dr T. L. Harris and associates in the *Proceedings of the Society for Experimental Biology and Medicine* in 1947. Forty young rats were placed on a diet deficient in both vitamins A and E, which is known to produce ulcers. After two weeks, all rats were given vitamin A but only half of them received vitamin E. After seven weeks the rats were examined for stomach lesions. One half, those on the high vitamin A, low vitamin E diet, had developed stomach ulcers. Not one animal in the group receiving vitamin E showed any sign of ulceration. We know that vitamin E strengthens muscular tissue and improves blood circulation. However, it also appears to help vitamin A function, in part by protecting it, so perhaps it is not surprising that vitamin E has remarkable healing properties in ulcerous conditions.

Other Curative Measures

The remaining curative measures are self-explanatory. They are:

(6) Avoid mixed, indiscriminate feeding.

(7) If you cannot eat a meal leisurely, in a state of mental and physical relaxation, it is better not to eat at all. The wise patient will cultivate the habit of having fifteen minutes' quiet repose before and after every meal, and he will have his meals at regular intervals.

(8) Omit all condiments.

(9) Cut out sugar. Never use saccharine. Substitute honey. By gradually reducing the amount of sweetening you like, you can easily cultivate a taste for unsweetened foods in a matter of weeks.

(10) With the introduction of such foods as wheat-germ, and the vitamins, you should have regular and adequate bowel movements without the use of

laxative pills or purgatives. Cut them out because they are dangerous irritants. If you still have any bowel trouble, take one or two teaspoons of molasses in warm water before going to bed.

(11) As we have seen, antacid and other alkaline powders are an unsound way of neutralizing stomach acidity. They offer a temporary respite from pain at the cost of making the condition worse. There is only one sound and certain way to cure excessive stomach acidity. Restore the proper acid-alkaline balance in your blood-stream by seeing that your diet consists of approximately 80 per cent of alkaline-forming foods and only about 20 per cent of acid-forming foods (see page 110 for details). If, in addition, you feed compatibly and generally follow the curative principles recommended, stomach acidity will plague you no more.

(12) Slow down the tempo of your life and cultivate the almost lost art of relaxation. Men who relax live longer—and it doesn't merely seem longer! To relax successfully you must make conscious and objective effort. Relax in the sun every day when possible, for fifteen to thirty minutes. The sun helps one to relax perfectly. It also helps to build good nerves—and good health. And make sure you get eight to nine hours' sleep at a regular retiring hour. The body repairs itself during sleep. There is no substitute for sleep, which Shakespeare described in *Macbeth* as 'Chief nourisher in life's feast'.

(13) Finally, by generally building up the health you also build up the resistance of the blood to noxious bacteria and virus invasions. This is of vital

importance to the ulcer sufferer because while his resistance is low, an ulcer is a breeding ground for harmful bacteria.

Dietary Suggestions for Treating Ulcers, Gastritis and Hiatus Hernia

The principle of these dietary suggestions is to buffer gastric acidity by providing several meals per day of palatable, non-irritating foods.

Foods that are allowed include milk, cream, prepared cereals (farina, cream of wheat, strained oatmeal, puffed rice, whole wheatflakes), gelatine, soup, potatoes, rice, polyunsaturated margarine, wholemeal bread, eggs, cooked fruits and vegetables, bananas (at certain times, see later), fruit juices, very lean meats (beef, lamb), fresh fish, cream or cottage cheese, custards, tapioca, rice or cornstarch pudding, plain cake made with wholewheat flours. Multivitamin supplementation is essential.

Foods to avoid include fried or highly seasoned food, spices, carbonated beverages, coffee, alcohol, meat broths, strong cheeses, coarse cereals or bread, raw fruits and vegetables (in the early stages of the complaint), rich desserts, pastry, nuts, olives and popcorn.

A typical sample bland diet is as follows:

Breakfast: Wheatgerm with milk or sugar; egg, bread with polyunsaturated margarine; jelly; milk; strained fruit or fresh fruit juices.

Lunch: Clear soup; lean meat; potato, rice or noodles; bread with polyunsaturated margarine; jelly; milk; strained fruit juices.

Dinner: Lean meat, fish or fowl; potato; two strained cooked vegetables; bread with polyunsaturated margarine; dessert; milk; strained fruit juices.

(Milk may be taken at any time between meals and at bedtime.)

Gastro-intestinal Tract Irritability

This diet is taken to spare the gastro-intestinal tract by frequent small feedings of easily digested low-residue nutrients. The content is sugars, milk, eggs, lean beef, lamb, fish or chicken, cooked refined cereals, enriched bread, polyunsaturated margarine, cottage or cream cheese, strained cooked fruits and vegetables (or juices), potatoes, bouillon, broth, clear soups, pasta, custards, dairy ice-cream, gelatine, milk puddings, plain cake.

For a low residue diet it is important to avoid highly seasoned or fried foods (to prevent irritation), whole or raw fruits and vegetables, wholegrain cereals and bread, bran, corn, dried legumes, port, excessive fat, nuts, jams and marmalade.

Strict Diet for Ulcer Sufferers

When ulcer symptoms are severe the following diet inhibits and neutralizes gastric acid secretions and relieves pain.

Step 1. Give 3 oz (90ml) of cold or chilled skimmed milk or milk drinks hourly between 7 am and 9 pm.

The drink may also be continued throughout the night if there is difficulty in sleeping.

Step 2. Continue the hourly milk feedings and gradually add egg and finely-ground cereal so that the patient is receiving egg instead of milk at 7 am and 7 pm. At 10 am, 1 pm and 4 pm, 3 oz (85g) of cooked cereal should replace the milk.

Step 3. A soft diet that provides essential nutrients in a form that is low in residue, well tolerated and easily digested. Suitable foods are strained soups and vegetables; fine wheat, corn or rice cereals; breads; cooked fruit (without skin or seeds); ripe bananas, grapefruit or orange sections; fresh fruit juices; potatoes; rice; ground beef; fish, fowl; eggs; cottage or cream cheese; milk; custards; gelatine; tapioca; milk puddings; ice-cream; plain cake.

Supplementary iron and other minerals, preferably as the well-absorbed amino acid chelates plus multivitamin supplements, are essential in these diets if the strict regime is continued for an extended time. Foods that must be avoided include raw fruits and vegetables, coarse breads and cereals, rich desserts, strong spices, veal, pork, all fried foods, nuts and raisins.

Diet and Vitamin Therapy for Peptic Ulcers and Acidity

Here is a suggested diet for stomach ulcer and acidity:

FIRST DAY

On rising: Glass of milk (to be sipped slowly, not drunk) with four B complex vitamin tablets.

Before breakfast: 1 vitamin A tablet, 1 B_1 (10mg) tablet, 1 B complex tablet (10mg potency), 1 vitamin C tablet (250mg), 1 vitamin E tablet or capsule (100mg), 1 teaspoonful of olive oil.

Breakfast: Three or more dessertspoons of a reputable brand of wheatgerm, and as much milk as you can tolerate without setting up a catarrhal condition. Soak the wheatgerm in milk (warm, if preferred) for five minutes before eating. If you prefer, the wheatgerm can be 'short cooked' for two or three minutes in milk. For flavouring or sweetening, use honey only. If this isn't enough for some appetites, the wheatgerm and milk may be followed by fresh or dried apricots and milk or cream. Alternatively a small quantity of grapes. As the condition improves, you can follow the wheatgerm and milk with ripe peaches, or grated apple and milk, or ripe or stewed apricots.
Note: Wheatgerm is not a starch, but a protein.

Mid-morning: Two teaspoons of brewer's yeast powder in a little milk. Alternatively, a thin slice of bread, butter and honey. If, however, you don't take the yeast at mid-morning, it should be taken at four o'clock or before retiring.

Before Lunch: The same vitamins as taken before breakfast, and 1 teaspoonful of olive oil.

Lunch: Two lightly poached eggs—no bread. Followed by grapes, if in season, or papaya. Do not eat bananas at this meal. Bananas are excellent by themselves or with other starch foods, but not with protein (eggs, meat, fish, cheese and nuts are protein).

Before the evening meal: The same vitamins as taken after breakfast with the addition of one pantothenic acid tablet and 1 teaspoonful of olive oil.

Evening meal: A plate of puréed vegetables—such as peas, beans, carrots, parsnips, spinach, pumpkin, cauliflower, etc. Without meat or fish, a plate of steamed vegetables is made more attractive by the addition of cheese sauce or butter sauce. Such a meal may be followed by the mild fruits, such as grapes, peaches, papaya, or banana-cream purée. If one has a juice extractor, carrot, cabbage, or beet-root juice are excellent for ulcers and health. Between meals, sip a glass of milk.

SECOND DAY

Pre-breakfast: Same as before.

Breakfast: Same as before or varied only as suggested.

Lunch: 3 oz (85g) cheese with celery. Alternatively, cheese and ripe peaches. Later on, when the ulcer has healed, make cheese and apple your standard luncheon, or a cheese salad.

Evening meal: Poached egg and vegetables—cooked as suggested. By way of a change, about every fourth night, a little grilled fish (but no potato or bread), followed by mild, ripe fruits only (no bananas).

The vitamin dosage, plus the olive oil, remains unchanged.

The Virtue of Potatoes

Dr L. J. Nye has pointed out that stomach ulcer is almost unknown in Ireland and he relates this to the fact that potatoes appear frequently in the Irish dietary. Dr Nye recommends that stomach ulcer patients take two potato meals a day. Potatoes mashed in milk can be taken by themselves as 'mid-meals'. Potatoes contain significant amounts of vitamin C and trace elements. Ulcer patients should ensure that the potatoes they eat are baked or boiled in their skins, as otherwise much of their nutritional value is lost in cooking. Although potatoes are classified as a starchy food, they must not be confused with the factory-processed and refined starches referred to elsewhere in this book, which are of dubious food value.

Coffee, Tea, Smoking and Aspirin

Coffee drinking excites the stomach acids into action when there is no work for them to do. A continual over-stimulation irritates the lining of the stomach and paves the way for stomach ulcers. Tea drinkers are advised to take weak tea with plenty of milk, and no sugar.

Excessive smoking destroys vitamin C in the body and thereby weakens the tissue forming the stomach. According to Dr W. J. McCormick, one cigarette depletes the body of 25mg of vitamin C.

The frequent use of aspirin, in powder or tablet form, is responsible for a good deal of stomach irritation, which can later develop into stomach ulcers. However, this can be reduced by ensuring that vitamin C is taken along with aspirin. For many years it has been known that aspirin causes over-excretion of vitamin C and hence its loss from the body, and may even contribute to its destruction. Vitamin C levels are reduced by chronic ingestion of aspirin as in some arthritic and rheumatic conditions. Now it has been proved in clinical trials that supplementary vitamin C improves the absorption of aspirin; replenishes the vitamin lost by the action of the drug; reduces the irritant action of aspirin on the gastric lining; enhances the pain-relieving properties of aspirin. Other non-steroidal anti-inflammatories used in arthritis have effects similar to those of aspirin. These too are reduced with supplementary vitamin C. It is important that vitamin C is taken at the same time as aspirin and the other drugs to obtain maximum benefit. The usual intake is 50-100mg vitamin C with each aspirin or other tablet.

After the Ulcer Heals
Dr D. T. Quigley advises those who have recovered from stomach ulcers to avoid canned and packaged foods, as they have been robbed of their nutrients by the application of high heat and long storage. He says that such foods are stale and worthless. He forbids his ulcer patients the use of cane sugar, which he calls a slow poison, also white flour products, which between them, constitute over 50 per cent of the food intake of the average person and thereby dilute whatever good, nourishing food the person eats by that amount.

The foods which Dr Quigley allows his patients after their stomach ulcers have healed are meat, milk, raw fruits and vegetables, eggs, unprocessed cheese, wholewheat foods and seafoods. He recommends that the patient consumes a minimum of a pound and half (680g) a day of raw fruits and vegetables, after the complete healing of the ulcer. Any fruit or vegetable that can be served raw, should be eaten raw. Salad vegetables should therefore be preferred to cooked vegetables. From three to six ounces (85-170g) of fresh meat should be eaten daily, cooked as 'rare' as is palatable. No salt meat is permissible, except ham and an occasional breakfast of bacon, and salty foods should be reduced to the minimum.

Dr Quigley says: 'The idea is to reject non-vitamin, non-mineral foods and keep this up for life ... Peptic ulcer is never caused by nervousness, it is associated with it. These persons are irritable and unstable, they are starved generally and specifically.' The reason for this is that 'the nerve disease and the ulcer both go back to a common cause: an over-supply of refined carbohydrates which causes a dangerous reduction of the vitamin and mineral concentration in the blood-stream. Stresses and strains and emotional upsets do not cause ulcer, but merely bring into more prominence conditions which already exist.'

After the ulcer has healed, make sure that you never get another stomach ulcer. You can do this by following Dr Quigley's advice and also by taking every day some brewer's yeast powder (for its vitamin B complex content), some vitamin A and D capsules, vitamin C (250mg) tablets and vitamin E (50mg) tablets or capsules.

Final Words

If any person cares to apply the thirteen curative principles previously recommended, and apply them intelligently and consistently, his stomach troubles should become a thing of the past in a matter of months. Improvement should be certain— except in those long-neglected cases in which the peritoneum has been perforated, or where some incurable ailment has developed. But it requires no small effort of will for the average person to break from his old feeding habits. Habit is so strong that when we change from bad to good feeding habits, the immediate reaction is that we feel the worse for it. But please don't misunderstand this. This phenomenon is simply due to the body reluctantly making its readjustments. Keep to the thirteen curative principles and in a few weeks a great improvement in your general health will make itself felt. The pain after meals should gradually ease and finally disappear. A new feeling of confidence and well-being will permeate body and mind. And, finally, victory over stomach ulcer should follow. But to be rid of a painful disease will not be your only satisfaction. The greater reward will be a far better standard of health and a new zest for life. No small return, you will agree, for the exercise of common sense, a few changes in your eating habits, and a little self-restraint.

Index